the
COSMO
BIKINI
DIET

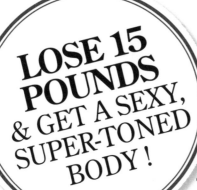

LOSE 15
POUNDS
& GET A SEXY,
SUPER-TONED
BODY !

the

COSMO
BIKINI
DIET

BY HOLLY C.
CORBETT
& THE EDITORS OF

COSMOPOLITAN

HEARST EDITIONS
NEW YORK

CONTENTS

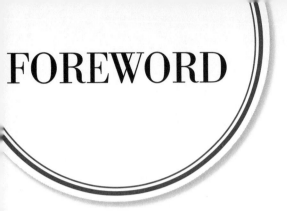

FOREWORD

At Cosmo, we aim to go beyond merely inspiring you to live a glamorous, sexy life by also arming you with the specific tools you need to actually achieve that life. Having a strong, toned body is one part of being your sexiest self, as is feeling healthy and energized.

That's why we created The Cosmo Bikini Diet. This isn't another yo-yo diet where you drop serious pounds only to regain them (and then some!) as soon as the program is over. Rather, our editors and team of experts specially developed a 12-week plan to help you shed pounds and get toned all over while nourishing your body and your mind with feel-good foods and fitness ideas.

The truth is, **reaching your happy weight** is not as much about hitting a number on the scale or size tag in your jeans as it is about feeling light and lean and strong. It's about getting there without abusing your body with extreme dieting and exercise. It's about eventually walking around—whether in a bikini or out!—with confidence, knowing that you are the healthiest you that you can be.

Feeling content and balanced on the inside is reflected in having a beautiful body on the outside. So here is what The Cosmo Bikini Diet is not: It's not a painful-to-follow, calorie-restrictive plan. It doesn't forbid your having all your favorite treats, such as chocolate or cocktails. It doesn't mean that you'll have to give up your social life and spend entire evenings at the gym in order to reach your weight-loss goals. Because depriving yourself is not sexy.

Rather, The Cosmo Bikini Diet is a realistic lifestyle program that makes healthy eating **easy and delicious**. It allows you to splurge on dates and hit up happy hours without feeling guilty. It makes exercising something you actually look forward to instead of dread, because we'll supply you with all different kinds of fun fitness ideas to keep workouts from feeling monotonous.

But it's so much more than even a food and fitness plan: This complete lifestyle program makes fitting in joy as much of a priority as sweat sessions and healthful eating.

The secret to getting your sexiest body means living a life that makes room for little pleasures, such as get-togethers with the girls or taking the time to get pumped by creating energizing playlists. The program is also about breaking ingrained habits and thought patterns that get in the way of attaining the bikini body you want, like tricks to overcome emotional eating.

In the pages that follow, you'll be armed with everything you need to succeed at getting the strong, toned body you've always dreamed of. But the real game changer is that you'll learn to improve your relationship with food, your body, and yourself. Here's to being your most fun, fearless, and sexy self on—and off—the beach!
—THE EDITORS OF COSMOPOLITAN

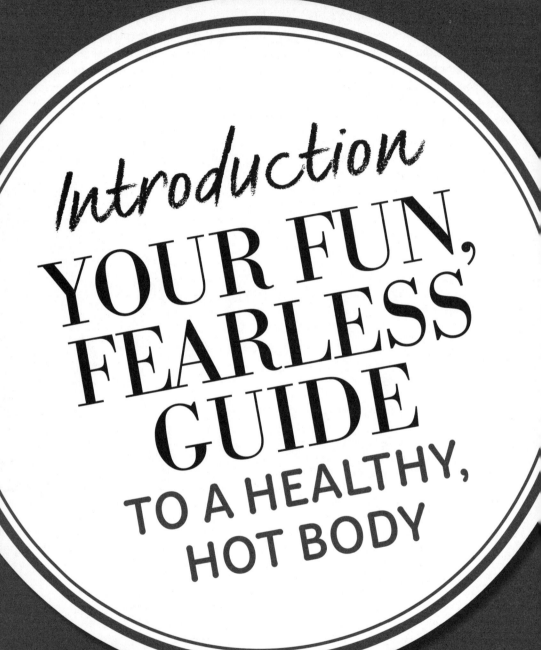

Introduction

YOUR FUN, FEARLESS GUIDE
TO A HEALTHY, HOT BODY

HOW TO USE THE COSMO BIKINI DIET

The Cosmo Bikini Diet is a weight-loss plan designed to get you slim and sexy all over without leaving you feeling unsatisfied, moody, and hungry—for real. In fact, it makes eating well and working out actually feel, well, enjoyable. That's why we think of it as an (*un*)diet.

This 12-week program gives you all the tools you need to drop pounds and get toned without cramping your lifestyle: Monthly real-world eating plans; Hot & Healthy Workouts that you can fit into even the busiest of schedules; ideas to up the feel-good moments in your day so you don't use food as a quick fix; and more. **You'll lose up to 15 pounds (or more) in 12 weeks without feeling deprived.**

The best part? You'll keep reaping the benefits of the Cosmo Bikini Diet long after the days of summer are gone by scoring a leaner, stronger body for life. That's because this new lifestyle we're showing you will be so energizing that you'll never want to go back to any bikini-body-sabotaging ways. You'll find that living the bikini body life is not only empowering, but also supereasy because we arm you with all the knowledge you'll need to succeed, such as how to whip up yummy and nourishing meals in no time; stay-slim secrets for eating out; and how to keep challenging your body with quick interval workouts to get tighter and more toned in less time.

This lifestyle program gives you delicious ideas for meals and snacks while showing you how to easily fit fitness into your already-full life. The Cosmo editors guide you every step of the way with week-by-week eating goals and monthly workout plans for a total of 12 weeks.

THE COSMO BIKINI DIET MEAL PLAN

Breaking old habits and making new ones take time—at least they do if you want them to stick. We won't be asking you to make big, overwhelming changes all at once, so we introduce only one new main eating goal each week along with advice on making it work in your daily life. **By the end of the program, you'll know and use all 12 goals (we think of them as our Cosmo Bikini Diet Secrets!) to get you your sexiest bikini body ever.**

We also won't inundate you with calorie counts or deprive you of your favorite things (a glass of red wine or a cocktail can still be your friend). We offer a detailed meal plan for each of the three months, specially designed for you by Molly Morgan, RD, board-certified sports specialist dietitian, the owner of Creative Nutrition Solutions, and author of *The Skinny Rules*. And if you prefer a less-structured approach, you can mix and match the breakfasts, lunches, dinners, or snacks whenever you need some flexibility. That's because each of the suggested meals and snacks has the ideal amount of calories, fat, protein, and healthy carbs for achieving and maintaining your best bikini body. That means you can swap in one snack for another snack, or stick to having the same breakfast all week long if you love it. Lunches and dinners have even more flexibility; either one can be swapped out for the other, since both lunches and dinners have roughly the same calories and mix of nutrients. You'll also get additional ideas, recipes, and foods tailored to each of the 12 Cosmo Bikini Diet Secrets in every chapter, so you can easily tweak your diet along the way. Plus, many days leave room for Flex Calories that you can spend as you like, be it on a glass of vino or a few squares of chocolate.

The Cosmo Bikini Diet Hot & Healthy Workout Plan

You won't have to log long hours at the gym to get a body you'll be proud to flaunt in a bikini. In fact, you'll exercise for only about 3 hours a week (some days for just 21 minutes tops)—and you get to take 2 whole days off to let your body recover. You'll switch up your routine every week, and advance your workout each month by increasing your weights, challenging your body to tone up faster while keeping you from getting bored. The weekends are reserved for moving in a way that feels like fun—not like another thing to check off your to-do list. You'll get weekly suggestions for new activities and fitness trends to ward off a workout rut and keep you motivated to reach your goals.

We've put together a team of top-notch trainers to create our unique fitness routine specially designed to get you the most banging bikini body in the least amount of time. Tracy Anderson, celebrity trainer for stars such as Gwyneth Paltrow and Madonna and creator of the Tracy Anderson Method, developed the 6-minute, body-part-specific toning sessions that you'll be doing twice a week. Barry Jay and Joey Gonzalez of Barry's Bootcamp (aka the "new DJs" of fitness) are famous for making workouts fun while earning you fast results. Their explosive interval training combined with targeted resistance moves is guaranteed to blast fat on your belly, butt, and thighs in just 30 minutes or less. They've coached celebs such as Kim Kardashian, Amanda Seyfried, Jessica Biel, and Katie Holmes to maintain their paparazzi-ready bikini bodies, and now they're helping *you* get smoking hot in time to hit the beach. It's like having your own personal celebrity trainers making house calls!

And it gets even better: No gym membership is required when it comes to the Cosmo Bikini Diet.

Here is the only gear you'll need to get started:
◆ A set of light weights (5 to 6 pounds), medium weights (8 pounds), and heavy weights (10 to 12 pounds)
◆ A jump rope
◆ A clock, stopwatch, or some sort of timer for keeping track of your sets (or the amount of time it takes to complete a specific number of reps of a specific move, such as bicep curls, before moving on to another move, such as squats).
◆ Supportive sneakers to wear for your Morning Cardio Blasts and strength and toning routines.

◆ One light and one heavy resistance band. Here are some guidelines for picking which bands are best for you:

- ◆ Resistance bands are color-coded to help differentiate between those that offer light tension and those that provide heavier tension. Generally, lighter-colored bands have less tension, while darker colors provide more tension, but keep in mind that each manufacturer color-codes its bands differently. Also, thicker bands offer more resistance than thinner bands.
- ◆ Light to medium bands are often color-coded green (and sometimes yellow). If you've never exercised before, you might want to start with the lightest band and then graduate to a band with medium tension. On the other hand, if you're already a fitness fanatic, you can start with an intermediate band before graduating to the most advanced band by the end of the program.
- ◆ The $5 resistance bands available at BarrysBootcamp.com are color-coded as follows: green for beginners, orange for medium tension, black for intermediate, and red for the most advanced option.

The Cosmo Bikini Diet (Un)Guilty Pleasures

Rewarding yourself is just as important as eating healthy and working out when it comes to reaching your happy weight. The weekly (Un)Guilty Pleasures are suggestions on ways to feel good rather than deprived. They're designed to help you take care of yourself—whether that means taking 20 minutes to eat lunch away from your desk or leaving the office at 5:30 to hit your favorite sample sale. When you're following the Cosmo Bikini Diet, we want you to enjoy your life to the fullest!

The COSMO BIKINI DIET PLEDGE

It's easy to tell yourself you're going to lose weight, but Cosmo makes actually doing it a no-brainer with the Cosmo Bikini Diet's weekly fitness and meal plans. Still, it takes making a commitment to yourself to succeed when embarking on any goal—whether it be taking control of your diet, your money, or your life. Stating your intention means you'll be more likely to stick with the program—and hop back on after those (inevitable) moments when you get off track. Start by signing and dating the Cosmo Bikini Diet Pledge, and be sure to add your own promises to yourself in the blank space at the end.

I WILL NOT OBSESS OVER CALORIES. Let's face it: Worrying about the calorie content of every forkful is about as much fun as seeing your ex with a new date and robs you of the pleasure of eating. Your body ultimately knows what it needs if you're listening to it: Counting calories obsessively blocks you from being able to truly tune in to your real hunger and fullness cues. After all, you have more important ways to use your brainpower (such as figuring out how to make your dream beach getaway happen) than mentally tallying the calorie count of every food you see. You'll be getting an ideal mix of nutrients by following the Cosmo Bikini Diet meal plan, so you can ditch the calorie worry and focus on how good your body—and mind—will feel.

I WILL SHOW SOME BODY LOVE. We're not saying you have to learn to love your cellulite, but bashing your body will only sabotage your motivation. Focus on something you love about your body (such as your breasts or your arms) rather than what you hate, and the pounds are sure to melt off faster and a whole lot easier.

I WILL PAY ATTENTION TO MY APPETITE AND PACE MY MEALS. When it comes to your daily meals, the goal is to simply stop when you are full (not when you have to unbutton your jeans!) and to eat roughly every 3 to 4 hours to keep your blood sugar levels from crashing and from sending you diving into a chocolate bar.

I WILL NOT PUNISH MYSELF FOR GOING OFF TRACK.

Gorging on ice cream may soothe you in the moment but may leave you with regret and feeling like the Goodyear Blimp immediately afterward. If you *do* go on a late-night pizza binge, simply note what triggered it (too much booze? a fight with your BF?) and then get back into your Bikini Diet routine in the morning. Remember, one day of overeating won't make you fat, and take the misstep as an opportunity to address the eating patterns you want to change. Beating yourself up over a mistake will only undermine your own good efforts.

I WILL DO SOMETHING THAT FEELS GOOD EVERY DAY. In

order to have a slim body, you must also feed your soul. An easy way to add a little fun and joy to your life is to make sure you treat yourself every single day. Put together a list of small, feel-good things that you can easily slip into your days and keep on hand for when you're feeling overwhelmed or just need a pick-me-up.

I WILL MAKE SLEEP A PRIORITY. Shedding pounds isn't only about

eating nourishing foods, but also about recharging your body with enough rest. Studies show people who skimp on sleep are more likely to be obese and have more belly fat, so aim to put your head on the pillow (late-night shows and iPhone off) at least 7 hours before your alarm is set to buzz.

I WILL CREATE A BIKINI BODY GOALS LIST. Is your goal to score

flatter abs, drop 10 pounds, or feel more confident in your clothes and comfortable in your skin? Whatever your aspiration, having a clear picture of what you want and writing it down before you begin helps turn it into reality. Take a picture of your list and keep it in your phone so you can glance at it whenever you need motivation to stick to your new healthy-living routine.

I WILL WRITE DOWN MY DAILY MEALS AND SNACKS IN A FOOD JOURNAL. Get a lightweight journal that's easy to throw in your

purse so you can keep track of what you're eating. Or try tracking your food in an app such as the one at MyFoodDiary.com. Keeping a food diary can help you double the amount of weight you lose, according to researchers at the Kaiser Permanente Center for Health Research. That's because recording what you eat makes you more likely to stay on track—you may think twice about reaching for a handful of M&Ms when you know you have to write it down. It also gives you a clear picture of your eating habits so you can better gauge what's working for you and what isn't.

And it's not just about the food you put in your mouth! Also use this journal as a place where you can write down how you were feeling when you ate (such as bored when you noshed on that bag of crackers before bed, or energized after eating a nutritious bowl of oats with bananas for breakfast). Your food journal can be a useful tool for slimming down because it also gives you the chance to look back and notice your emotional-eating triggers so you can have a plan of attack ready for the next time.

I WILL RECORD MY WEEKLY MEASUREMENTS IN THE "SUCCESS TRACKER" SECTION. You'll find a spot to write down your weight and bust/waist/hip measurements at the end of each chapter so you can easily watch your progress over the 12-week program. Be sure to enter your starting measurements below so that you have your baseline to compare to. (The correct way to measure your waist is to place a measuring tape around the narrowest part of your natural waist—usually just above your belly button. The best way to measure your hips is to place the measuring tape around your hips at the widest part of your butt.) This is also a place to make notes about how you feel during each phase (such as more energized, less bloated, more confident, etc.). Another motivational trick: Watch yourself shrink—literally. With the FITEO app (free at the iTunes App Store), you'll take a daily pic of a specific body area, then watch your weight-loss and muscle-sculpting progress via a time-lapse video for serious slimspiration.

I WILL SURROUND MYSELF WITH HEALTHY BIKINI BODY MOTIVATORS. Try hanging out more often with women whose healthy attitudes inspire you to get in shape (and less often with those who starve themselves or hate on their bodies). Sweating it out next to a friend who is motivated to fit in fitness is contagious. Bonus if her body is strong, healthy, and rocks a bikini, because seeing another woman who has mastered a healthy lifestyle will remind you that you can do it, too.

I WILL _____

_____

_____

_____

_____

_____

I WILL _____

_____

_____

_____

_____

I WILL _____

_____

_____

_____

_____

I WILL _____

_____

_____

_____

_____

I WILL _____

_____

_____

_____

_____

Signed by: _____ **Date:** _____

SUCCESS TRACKER

Starting Measurements

Weight _____

Waist _____

Chest _____

Hips _____

My Happy Weight Goal

Weight _____

Waist _____

Chest _____

Hips _____

Month 1

THE SKINNY

STARTING THE COSMO BIKINI DIET

HOW MUCH WEIGHT WILL YOU LOSE?

Getting your sexiest bikini body is easier than ever: Cosmo has done all the meal planning for you so you don't have to stress about what to eat or count every little calorie. This 12-week plan starts with a Jump-Start Week that sets you up to lose as many as 3 pounds in the first week, followed by a healthy 1 to 2 pounds a week after that. You can expect to drop up to 15 pounds or more.

The Jump-Start Week will teach you about portion control and allows about 1,500 calories a day, enough to help you feel full and satisfied as well as ensure that you see immediate results to keep you motivated. In the following weeks, we've added 150 daily Flex Calories (see page 19) to bring you to 1,600 to 1,650 calories daily. All the special weekly meal plans are nutritionally balanced and target Cosmo's 12 Bikini Diet Secrets.

Each week is set up to help you tackle and learn new ways of eating right. And while the purpose of the Cosmo Bikini Diet plan is, of course, to get you Bikini Diet–ready, it's also about adopting a healthy lifestyle that you can maintain for life.

Each meal and snack has a perfect mix of core nutrients:
◆ 50 percent of calories (about 200 grams per day) from carbohydrates
◆ 20 percent of calories from protein (about 80 grams per day)
◆ 30 percent of calories from fat (53 grams or fewer per day)
◆ About 35 grams of filling fiber

Keep in mind that the number of calories that your body needs varies greatly based on height, weight, and how much you're working out. For example, if you're doing more exercise than outlined in this book—like training for a half marathon—you will need more calories in order to fuel your workouts. If you're doing less exercise than the Cosmo Bikini Diet recommends, you may need fewer calories.

The ideal rate of weight loss is 1 to 2 pounds per week (though you'll probably lose at least 3 in the Jump-Start Week). After a few weeks, if you find you're losing weight more slowly, then you can up your exercise (try fitting in additional 15-minute Morning Cardio Blasts on your "off" days) or reduce your calorie intake slightly (skipping the Flex Calories is an option during any week of the plan if you find the scale gets stuck).

If you're losing weight more quickly, you'll need to adjust your overall calorie intake, because dropping too much weight too fast is not healthy and ultimately undermines your diet efforts. (Try adding an extra snack into your day.) That's because dropping weight too fast (such as 4 pounds a week) means you're probably losing mostly water weight and muscle mass. But muscle mass is vital to help increase metabolism and make you looked toned. And melting the real bikini body saboteur—fat—takes time. Plus, deprivation diets where you lose a lot of weight quickly can send your body into starvation mode, so you're more apt to store nutrients as fat. Deprivation diets are also impossible to sustain, so you won't be able to hold on to your bikini body for long. And isn't your goal to look hot for the long haul rather than slim down only to pack on the pounds again shortly after?

The Meal Plan

Each monthly meal plan offers breakfasts, lunches, dinners, snacks, and Flex Calories. Molly Morgan, RD, has created the meal plans with a mix-and-match approach to give you flexibility, allowing you to choose which meal options work best for you! You'll find the easy-to-prepare recipes in Chapter 14. If for some reason you can't follow the specific meal plan for a particular day or you're choosing foods from restaurants (find the nutritional information online before you dine!) or are traveling . . . good news! You can still stick to the diet by sticking to these guidelines. Here's the rough breakdown:

The meals
◆ Breakfast (250 calories)
◆ Lunch (450 calories)
◆ Dinner (450-500 calories)
◆ Snacks (two a day for 300 calories total)
◆ Flex Calories (150 calories)

These calorie and nutrient counts stay the same throughout all the monthly meal plans (except for the Jump-Start Week, which does not have any Flex Calories). This approach gives you ultimate flexibility to pick and choose which meals and snacks work best for you. For example, all breakfasts have roughly the same number of calories and nutrients. Don't feel like an egg? Then swap out one day's egg-based breakfast for another day's that features a smoothie or oatmeal or something else that you're more in the mood for. The same goes for snacks all having the same number of calories. Since both lunches and dinners have roughly equal calorie and nutrient counts, you can even swap in a lunch for a dinner and vice versa. (Breakfasts have fewer calories, so you can swap only one breakfast for another in order to stick to the plan.) You'll always be eating the right mix of nutrients and calories to help you slim down!

Snacks: Snacks are a Bikini Diet staple because they tame your appetite to ward off bingeing later on. Don't think of snacks as an indulgence: Rather, they are diet essentials to stop hunger and keep your metabolism revved throughout the day! Each meal plan includes about 300 calories coming from snacks, split between two snacks per day (or roughly 150 calories each). We'll give you plenty of ideas, and you can swap in your favorite snacks if you're not into a snack suggested on another day in the meal plan.

Flex Calories: These 150 calories are your daily indulgence (except during the Jumpstart week) to "spend" however you like. For the meal plan days that include a specific dessert option, we're simply suggesting how to spend those 150 fun calories—but you can opt to have a glass of wine or a serving of chips or a cookie instead, if that's what you want most (just don't have both!).

If you don't use your Flex Calories one day, you can save them up over 2 or 3 days for an upcoming event or night out (although it's best to use them evenly throughout the week to keep your calorie intake consistent).

The Deal With Drinks

Between Meals: Sip on water

Sipping on water throughout the day is a skinny secret, because staying hydrated keeps you from mistaking thirst for hunger and overeating. The good news: There are plenty of ways to keep water calorie free but not boring. Try these tricks:

◆ **Fruit and veggies:** Add sliced cucumbers, oranges, or strawberries to water for a flavor twist.

◆ **Herbs:** Mint and lavender makes plain old tap water taste fit for a spa.

◆ **Seltzer water:** The fizz makes your water feel fancy. Opt for naturally flavored types like lemon, blackberry, or pomegranate.

◆ **Swanky ice cubes:** Try adding basil, berries, vanilla extract, or other flavorings to your ice cube trays when freezing, and let them melt into a tall glass of water for an extra kick.

With Breakfast: Coffee or tea and juice

Coffee and tea are essentially calorie free! Minimize added calories from sweeteners: Each teaspoon of honey, agave, or sugar has about 16 calories. It may not sound like a lot, but 16 calories can pile up to unwanted pounds in a hurry if you're having a few mugs a day. For example, if you have three cups every morning, that's about 5 added pounds' worth of calories over the course of a year! Try slowly taming your sweet tooth by cutting the amount of sugar or artificial sweeteners you use in half. (Just because artificial sweeteners are calorie free doesn't mean they're good for your bikini body! See page 138 for more on fake sugars.) See if you can eliminate them completely by the end of the diet.

You can also use your Flex Calories for splurging at, say, coffee meetings, where you may want to order something more interesting than sipping it black. Just beware of fancy drinks that are hidden calorie bombs! A Caramel Ribbon Crunch Frappuccino from Starbucks has 560 calories and 18 grams of fat, which more than blows your Flex Calorie daily limit—and costs you even more calories than your lunch or dinner (see more about how to eat healthy while eating out in Chapter 9).

Watch out also for fruit juice (see "The Real Deal on the Juicing Trend" on page

142). An 8-ounce glass can have 150 or more calories, which quickly spends much of the 250 calories allotted for breakfast. If you're a juice girl, you can always opt to have 8 ounces of 100% fruit juice as your Flex Calories for the day.

With Lunch and Dinner: Milk or a Milk Substitute or Seltzer Water

Some of the meals incorporate low-fat milk or a milk substitute. The reason we include milk with lunch and dinner is that the beverage is filled with bone-strengthening nutrients like calcium, magnesium, and vitamin D. When choosing milk, always opt for 1% (low-fat) or fat-free milk. When going for a milk substitute like almond milk, skip the sugary types and choose one that's fortified with calcium and vitamin D. Here are some choices:

- 1 cup fat-free milk: 90 calories
- 1 cup unsweetened almond milk: 40 calories
- 1 cup original almond milk: 60 calories
- 1 cup original soy milk: 90 calories
- 1 cup rice milk: 120 calories

The meal plans are designed to allow for 1 to 2 cups of milk or milk alternative per day. The calories for any drink listed in the meal plan are included in the total calorie count. So don't stress about gulping extra calories if one night's dinner calls for a cup of milk—we have it covered! Many meals incorporate calorie-free drinks, like unsweetened tea or seltzer water, which you can swap for another zero-calorie beverage. Keep in mind that adding in a glass of milk or juice or wine when it's not listed for that meal in the plan will up your daily calorie intake. If you want to have a drink that's not included in the meal plan, just be sure to bank that drink as your Flex Calories for the day.

Alcohol

We leave room in each meal plan to enjoy a glass of wine or a cocktail if you feel like it, because we give you Flex Calories that you can spend any way you want. And if there's a night when you know you're going to want two or three drinks, you can save your Flex Calories from two or three other days so you don't overdo your calorie limit. (Try to avoid banking more than 3 days of Flex Calories at a time so you don't fall into a cycle of binges.)

TAKING YOUR "EARNED" DAY OFF

Each week includes six daily meal plans plus one day off. Rather than looking at this day as a "cheat" day, look at it as an "earned" day for sticking to the healthy eating and fitness program that week. It's up to you to design your ideal earned eating day by fueling up on high-fiber, nutrient-dense foods as outlined in the Bikini Diet eating plan, all while allowing a little wiggle room to reward yourself with a favorite food—be it a hot fudge sundae, curly fries, or sangria. If you don't want to design your own day, simply repeat one of the days from the week's meal plans, but allow yourself a favorite treat.

Remember, the Cosmo Bikini Diet is super easy because all our meals and snacks stick to the above guidelines, so you can eat a lunch option from Day 1 of the meal plan even though you're on Day 4, and you won't throw off your calorie count or nutrients. The beauty of being able to interchange all meals and snacks however you'd like is that you can customize the diet to be the perfect fit for you.

The Cosmo Bikini Diet Meal Plan Weeks 1–4

Any day is a good day to start the Bikini Diet, but pick the day that works best for you based on your own schedule. Maybe Sunday makes the most sense because you have more time to shop and purge your cupboards of tempting junk food. It's a good idea to start on a day when you can make a batch of nourishing meals or portion out nutritious snacks for the week ahead. By starting your week healthy, you'll be even more motivated to make real changes and stick with 'em all week long.

Plan each week in advance by stocking up on healthy snacks and figuring out which day you'll take off. Your earned day off doesn't have to be the same day every week, but map it out ahead of time. You'll find it easier to stick to your healthy eating plan when you can look forward to the day when you can splurge. For example, one week you may have a date on Saturday night and want that to be your earned day, so you can savor a decadent dinner, while the next Thursday may be happy hour with the girls, so you know you'll want to have an extra cocktail or two on that night.

After you map out your eating routine for the next 7 days, draft your shopping list and go shopping so that you have all of the ingredients on hand to put the plan into action. (See the shopping lists in Chapter 13.) Pretty soon, planning ahead will become second nature and easy to do. See the chart on the next page for a cheat sheet of this month's meal plan, and see page 163 for recipes.

BIKINI DIET MEAL PLA

day	BREAKFAST	SNACK	LUNCH
1	Cereal w/sliced almonds, milk & berries (p. 163); coffee or tea	Veggies w/ hummus (p. 168)	Tuna fish salad sandwich (p. 164); apple; seltzer wate
2	Scrambled egg on toast (p. 163); berries; coffee or tea	Low-fat cottage cheese w/ kiwi fruit (p. 169)	Black bean soup w/ whole wheat baguette (p. 164); apple and cheese; unsweetened tea
3	Whole wheat English muffin w/cheese spread and blackberries (p. 163); coffee or tea	Dark chocolate w/ sliced strawberries (p. 169)	Chicken & veggie wrap (p. 164); spinach salad (p. 164) w/ Healthy Balsamic Dress (p. 165); seltzer water
4	Apple cinnamon oatmeal (p. 163); coffee or tea	100-calorie pack of guacamole w/ veggies (p. 169)	Veggie pita (p. 165); cottag cheese; fruit; seltzer water
5	Whole wheat waffle w/nut butter & sliced banana (p. 163); coffee or tea	1 large hard-boiled egg w/ 10 wheat crackers (p. 169)	Italian flatbread (p. 165) w/ cherry tomatoes; fruit; wate
6	Mexican breakfast scramble (p. 164); coffee or tea	Applesauce & almonds (p. 169)	Veggie & chicken salad w/ Greek yogurt (p. 165); fruit; seltzer water
7	EARNED DAY ⟶ (page 34)		

WEEKLY AVERAGE DAILY NUTRITION FACTS: About 1,500 calories for the Jump-Start Week, plus 150 Flex Calories for the following weeks for about 1,650 calories total, 53 g total fat, 15 g saturated fat, 0 g trans fat, 17 g monou saturated fat, 6 g polyunsaturated fat, 242 m cholesterol, 2,148 mg of sodium, 174 g carb hydrates, 30 g fiber, 74 g sugar, 90 g protein

HEAT SHEET

NACK	DINNER	FLEX CALORIES*
eek yogurt w/honey d almonds (p. 168)	Chicken tagine w/olives (p. 166); apricot-herb couscous (p. 166); asparagus (p. 167); milk or milk substitute	150 calories to spend as you like
pcorn w/ Spice Salt (p. 169)	Flank steak or filet mignon w/ sautéed onions (p. 167); baked sweet potato (p. 167); green beans (p. 167); milk or milk substitute	150 calories to spend as you like
ed apricots & sun- wer seeds (p. 169)	Veggie-avocado burger on tomato bun (p. 167); fruit; zucchini; milk or milk substitute	150 calories to spend as you like
-skim cheese k; pear (p. 169)	Steak salad (p. 168) w/garlic toast (p. 168); milk or milk substitute	150 calories to spend as you like
tachios & dried nberries (p. 169)	Grilled salmon (p.168) w/ mashed cauliflower (p. 168); sliced mango; milk or milk substitute	Berries w/vanilla yogurt (p. 169) or 150 calories to spend as you like
ery w/peanut ter & raisins (p. 169)	Butternut squash soup w/ cheesy tomato wrap (p. 168); milk or milk substitute	150 calories to spend as you like

tio of calories from carbohydrates, protein, d fat: 50% carbohydrates, 23% protein, and % fat.

*REMEMBER TO SKIP THE FLEX CALORIES during the Jump-Start Week.

HOT & HEALTHY WORKOUTS WEEKS 1-4

The key to toning up fast is to work out smarter, not harder. It sounds counterintuitive, but spending hours on the StairMaster won't transform your body. "Working out too hard doesn't help much with fat loss because you burn fat more efficiently at a lower heart rate, and doing more than 30 minutes of cardio may cause you to burn metabolism-boosting muscle," says Paul "PJ" James, certified personal trainer and author of *Take It Off, Keep It Off.*

You'll be following this plan every week:
1. A 15-minute Morning Cardio Blast routine, 4 to 5 days
2. A 6-minute targeted toning routine, twice a week
3. A 20-minute Total-Body Strength Circuit routine, twice a week
4. Feel-Good Fitness, once a week
5. Rest and recover, twice a week

In each of the first 4 weeks, we feature a new 15-minute morning cardio routine from Barry's Bootcamp which you'll do before you even think about eating breakfast. A study in the *British Journal of Nutrition* finds that people who work out in the morning on an empty stomach burn 20 percent more fat than those who eat breakfast before their sweat session. While we give you a different routine each week, if you like one in particular, you can opt to stick to that. The important thing is doing high-intensity intervals for 15 minutes in the morning to get your heart pumping! You'll do these four to five times a week.

The Cosmo Bikini Diet is designed to torch calories while building metabolism-boosting muscle. Quick, body-part-specific toning workouts (6 minutes each) from celebrity trainer Tracy Anderson target specific body areas, such as your butt or your thighs, to get you toned all over. You'll do these twice a week.

Total-Body Strength Circuits are guaranteed to melt belly fat and come from the guys at Barry's Bootcamp, who are famous for sculpting bikini bodies fast. These routines will take 20 minutes, and you'll do them twice a week.

To keep exercise fun, we've got a Feel-Good Fitness Day every week when you'll look for new ways to get moving, such as taking a hip-hop dance class or trying karate. Not sure what to do? We'll give you fresh ideas for sweating it out and you can always repeat one of the other daily exercise plans if you prefer—but try to move your body for at least 45 minutes, such as by adding in a brisk walk to one of the 21-minute workout days.)

Even the two nonconsecutive days of rest have a purpose: To let your muscles recover to maximize your results.

Since no one's schedules are exactly the same, pick whichever days work best for you to do any of the suggested workouts. Other than the Morning Cardio Blasts, just avoid doing the same type of strength and toning workouts back-to-back on 2 consecutive days. That's because you want to give those muscles that you just worked time to repair. You'll find instructions for all the routines in Chapter 15.

HOT & HEALTHY
WORKOUT CHEAT SHEET

WEEKS 1-4

You'll find instructions for all the routines in Chapter 15.

DAY	WORKOUT	MINUTES
1	Morning Cardio Blast (pages 188, 195, 198, 201)	15
	Tracy Anderson's Toning Routine (pages 188, 196, 199, 202)	6
	TOTAL WORKOUT TIME	**21**
2	Morning Cardio Blast (pages 188, 195, 198, 201)	15
	Barry's Bootcamp Total-Body Strength Circuit (pages 190, 195, 198, 202)	20
	TOTAL WORKOUT TIME	**35**
3	Rest and recover!	
4	Morning Cardio Blast (pages 188, 195, 198, 201)	15
	Tracy Anderson's Toning Routine (pages 188, 196, 199, 202)	6
	TOTAL WORKOUT TIME	**21**
5	Morning Cardio Blast (pages 188, 195, 198, 201)	15
	Barry's Bootcamp Total-Body Strength Circuit (pages 190, 195, 198, 202)	20
	TOTAL WORKOUT TIME	**35**
6	Rest and recover!	
7	Morning Cardio Blast (Optional) (pages 188, 195, 198, 201)	15
	Feel-Good Fitness day (pages 194, 197, 200, 203)	30-45
	TOTAL WORKOUT TIME	**45-60**

CHAPTER ONE

MIND YOUR PORTIONS

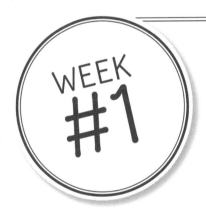

WEEK #1

THE LOWDOWN While paying attention to portions seems like common sense, it's all too easy to get distracted and polish off a whole bag of pita chips with a container of hummus while watching a *Scandal* marathon. (We'll admit it; we're obsessed!) Even healthy food choices can keep you from getting the bikini body you crave if you're not eating mindfully and end up noshing too much.

This week's goal is to become more aware of what portion sizes really look like, because you may be seriously underestimating how much you eat. Measuring your servings helps retrain your brain (and stomach!) to know that you probably don't need as much food as you may have grown accustomed to eating. This is also the first week you'll be keeping your food diary—an important tool to understand portion sizes. Noting portion sizes also makes you more aware of the difference between hunger and emotional eating. Simply by making this little diet tweak—going for the right portion sizes—you'll be able to shed up to 3 pounds this first week without changing any of your other eating habits!

Turn to the Meal Plan Cheat Sheet on page 22 for specifics on what to eat. While you're focusing on portion control this week, eliminate the Flex Calories to speed your weight loss for this first Jump-Start Week. Be sure to drink plenty of water to help keep hunger under control. For more detailed portion and food-prep info, turn to Chapter 14, page 162.

This chapter offers:
◆ a simple guide on how to eyeball serving sizes so you won't ever have to mess with food scales
◆ six effortless tricks for eating less
◆ the top 11 secrets to dieting success
◆ upbeat song suggestions for your exercise playlist
◆ an easy move for sleeping yourself skinny (no joke!)
◆ and more!
Ready, set, start losing!

THE SHOCKING TRUTH ABOUT PORTION SIZES

Turns out, what we think is one portion or one serving is way bigger. It's as though we've unconsciously supersized what a normal portion should look like. As a result, we're eating much more than we think. For example, many cereal boxes say a serving is a measly ¾ cup (about a handful and a half). It's way too easy to pour triple that amount into your bowl and unknowingly consume an additional 200 calories. Start to pay attention to the portion sizes stated on packaged foods. And if you're not into weighing or measuring your food, use this simple guide to train your eyes to recognize what a portion size *really* looks like.

PROTEIN: A serving of meat of fish is about 3 to 4 ounces, about the size of an iPhone. One egg or three whites also equals a serving of protein.

CARBS: A single portion of most carbs, such as rice or grains, is about the size of your fist. Here is how to eyeball a portion of different types of carbs:
A cupped handful = ¾ cup grains, such as cereal and oatmeal
CD case = A 1-slice serving of bread (½ a bagel is also a serving)
Computer mouse = ½ cup pasta

FATS: A serving size is usually an ounce or a tablespoon.
One die = A tablespoon of oil, butter, margarine, or fatty spreads like cream cheese
Golf ball = Two tablespoons equals a serving of peanut butter, sunflower seeds, or sesame seeds
Shot glass = One serving of nuts is an ounce. You can eat about 30 pistachios for the

same number of calories you'd nosh with 10 cashews or almonds—but they'll all fit into a shot glass for easy measuring.

THE COSMO BIKINI DIET GUIDE TO PORTION CONTROL
Follow these six simple tricks to eat less without feeling like you're even trying.

1 **Downsize your plates.** Anyone who has ever polished off a family-sized bag of chips or entire bowl of bar nuts on her own knows that we tend to finish what's on our plates rather than eat the amount that our bodies actually need. If you shrink the size of your dishes by a quarter—such as going from a 12-inch plate to a 9-inch plate—you'll slash your portions without feeling deprived. The research backs it up: People serving themselves ice cream in larger bowls ate 31 percent more than those eating from smaller bowls—and both groups reported feeling full, according to the *American Journal of Preventive Medicine*.

2 **Divide and conquer.** A stay-slim trick may be as simple as dividing food into smaller packages. Study participants who were given 24 individually wrapped cookies ate them in an average of 24 days, while those who received a box of 24 without the partitions polished them off in just 6, according to the *Journal of Marketing Research*. Partitioning food keeps you from eating larger portions, because stopping to open another package forces you to pay attention to how much you're actually downing. But before you stock up on bulk boxes of 100-calorie-pack treats, know that partitions may lose their effect over time if ripping into another package becomes a routine task.

3 **Choose a cozy restaurant.** Got a big date night coming up? Go ahead and enjoy—so long as the ambience is romantic. Diners eating in restaurants that have soft music and soft lighting eat 18 percent less overall—or about 175 fewer calories—than those in brighter, noisier joints, according to a study in the journal *Psychological Reports*. Bonus: Diners also report enjoying their meals more. Experts speculate that eating in a relaxed environment helps you slow down and savor your food so you end up consuming less overall. You can do it yourself at home by playing your most chill iPod mix and lighting some candles.

4 **Slow down when you chew.** Women who chewed at least 20 times before swallowing ate up to 70 calories less at mealtime, according to the *American Journal of Clinical Nutrition*. Another study in the journal *Appetite* found that people who chewed each mouthful of their lunch for 30 seconds noshed less than half as many sweets later in the afternoon compared to those who chewed for less time. Since it takes 20 to 30 minutes for your body to register that you're full, some researchers think slow eating

lets you get to the point when you feel satisfied on fewer calories. Others speculate that chewing slowly helps you savor and enjoy your food more so you eat less overall.

5 **Leave a few forkfuls on your plate.** Restaurant dishes are up to 250 percent larger than a normal portion size, so you can save up to 500 calories just by leaving a quarter of the meal on your plate. You can also easily cut portions at home by getting into the habit of leaving just a few forkfuls on your plate to save hundreds of calories over the course of the day.

6 **Try the 15-minutes delay.** Giving in to cravings won't sabotage your bikini body—so long as you stick to petite portions like a few bites of a brownie or handful of fries. If you think there's no way that a couple of mouthfuls could possibly satisfy your sweet tooth or salty cravings, think again: A study in the journal *Food, Quality and Preference* discovered that people served large snack portions downed a whopping 77 percent more calories than those served smaller portions—but both groups reported an equal drop in their hunger pains. Another portion control trick? Waiting 15 minutes also cut cravings for both groups. The no-deprivation secret to portion control may be to go ahead and indulge in a few bites of a decadent salty or sweet treat, and then walk away or do something else to distract yourself for 15 minutes. Chances are you'll feel satisfied and not need to polish off the entire treat.

STAR-SPIRATION FROM SINGER-SONG-WRITER KELLY CLARKSON

"I was working with a trainer, and she said, 'You'd be amazed the amount of weight you can drop by halving your portions. I know it sounds crazy, but do it for two weeks and watch what happens.' I just cut back my portions, I stopped eating late at night, and I work out a little more than I used to, and I literally dropped 18 pounds in a month."

THE TOP 11 TRICKS FOR DIET SUCCESS

The success rates of most diets are less than 5 percent, because restrictive eating plans or hard-core fitness regimens just aren't sustainable. Is a life without wine and chocolate worth living? Do you really want to spend 2 hours a day on the treadmill? We think not. Reaching your happy weight starts with changing your mind-set about exercise and food—and having your sexiest body will be easier than ever if you follow these tried-and-true lifestyle tricks.

1 **Eat for volume.** While portion control is important, you don't have to eat like a bird to lose weight. A good rule is to always fill half your plate at lunch and dinner with vegetables (or low-sugar fruits) to quickly cut down on the room you have for higher-calorie and fatty foods. That's because a quarter cup of veggies is about 10 calories, while the same amount of starches may bank you 50 calories, so you can eat bigger portions without breaking your calorie bank (see the list of fruits and veggies on page 158). And start your meal with a salad or cup of broth-based (not creamy!) soup so you'll fill up faster on fewer calories without feeling hungry.

2 **Find a fitness frenemy.** You've probably heard having a gym buddy is good for your workout. Turns out, exercising with someone who can one-up you (she's a little faster, a little stronger) is even better: Women worked out twice as long with a partner they were competitive with than they did when sweating solo, research from Kansas State University shows. The researchers suspect that fit friends inspire us to bring our A-game.

3 **Think yourself slim.** To curb a nighttime binge, try thinking back to what you had for dinner. Study participants asked to recall their last meal before doing a taste test ate about one-third fewer cookies than those who were asked about their morning commute, finds a study in *Physiology & Behavior*. That's because remembering what you ate activates your brain's hippocampus, which may play a role in decision making to help you say no to consuming extra calories. So try mentally picturing everything you had for lunch (no cheating!) before making your routine afternoon vending-machine visit. You may decide you don't need those potato chips after all!

4 **Limit your food choices.** Keeping a lot of different foods in your kitchen may make it harder to avoid temptation. If you want to ward off overeating, stock your cupboards and lunch bag with a smaller variety of healthy foods, because having too many choices may actually sap your willpower. After all, decisions take energy, and having many options (cereal, popcorn, chips, crackers, nuts or granola bars) challenges your self-control. So stay away from those all-you-can-eat buffets and stick to your go-to meal—you'll conserve your willpower for those times when it *really* counts (like when your cubicle mate brings in her addictive brownies).

10 ENERGIZING SONGS TO CRANK UP YOUR EXERCISE

Don't underestimate the feel-good benefits of downloading a new playlist before your next sweat session. Rocking out not only helps distract you from your huffing and puffing, but it also makes you feel more excited, say researchers at Brunel University in the United Kingdom. Different tempos of music have stronger effects for different types of workouts. The best motivator for strength training is between 120 and 140 beats per minute (bpm), such as heavy metal or hip-hop. Dance remixes between 147 to 160 beats per minute may work best for cardio sessions, such as running. Crank up your workout by adding these songs to your playlist, or find out the bpm of your favorite songs at bpmdatabase.com and customize your own.

1. "Super Bass" by Nicki Minaj (145 bpm)
2. "California Gurls" by Katy Perry with Snoop Dogg (125 bpm)
3. "Walk This Way" by Aerosmith (107 bpm)
4. "Hey Ya!" by Outkast (160 bpm)
5. "On the Floor" by Jennifer Lopez featuring Pitbull (150 bpm)
6. "California Love" by 2Pac and Dr. Dre (91 bpm)
7. "Don't Stop the Music" by Rihanna (122 bpm)
8. "Single Ladies (Put a Ring On It)" by Beyoncé (130 bpm)
9. "Tik Tok" by Ke$ha (120 bpm)
10. "Stronger" by Kanye West (104 bpm)

5 **Drink up.** Sometimes hunger is triggered by thirst rather than your body actually needing more calories. Try drinking a glass of water before eating. You may find your appetite quickly diminishes.

6 **Make it spicy.** A little sprinkling action may be all it takes to lose weight. In fact, people who added flavorings to their food shed an average of 30 ½ pounds, or nearly 15 percent of their body weight, after just 6 months, finds a study from the Smell & Taste Treatment and Research Foundation in Chicago. Seasonings may make bland-but-healthy foods, such as tofu and vegetables, taste better, so people are likelier to fill up on those lower-calorie options instead of craving fattier dishes. Try adding onion powder or chili pepper flakes to vegetables or topping sweet treats with cocoa powder or cinnamon to feel more satisfied and to slim down.

7 **Keep tabs on what goes in your mouth.** Remember: Studies show keeping a food diary helps you lose weight because it prevents mindless eating. If you're not into carrying around a journal, try texting or e-mailing yourself right after you nosh. Recording what you eat immediately makes it more accurate, because you're less likely to forget and underestimate calories if you try to write it all down at the end of the day. Turn it into a kind of game with yourself by tracking your food in an app such as the one mentioned in the Bikini Diet Pledge at MyFoodDiary.com (see page 13).

8 **Cook at home.** Eating at home can lead to losing weight in more ways than one. Besides avoiding those supersized restaurant portions, cooking burns about 90 calories in 30 minutes (based on a 150-pound person). Taking a cooking class can also help you break free from a food rut. Many places offer basic cooking seminars now, especially larger health-food stores such as Whole Foods.

9 **Know before you go.** Check out the nutrition information found on many restaurant chains' websites before you eat out. Diners who saw nutrition information before selecting their meals ate an average of 52 fewer calories, according to the *American Journal of Public Health*. Moreover, you'll be able to make smarter meal choices. Instead of having Chili's Steak and Portobello Fajitas for 1,130 calories, you can choose Chili's Classic Chicken Fajitas for just 360 calories—a savings of almost 800!

10 **Log off Facebook.** If you can't get rid of your belly fat, you might want to set a limit on the amount of time you spend browsing social-networking sites to free you up to get off the couch. Research finds that the more time you log on Facebook and Twitter, the less time you spend on physical activity—and the less likely you are to play team sports. The flipside: Using social media for weight-loss support can actually help shrink your middle. That means sending diet status updates like "I avoided eating a pastry this morning at a breakfast meeting! I did have a skim mocha without

whipped cream . . . not too bad." Every 10 diet-related posts to Twitter equaled a drop in weight of about half a percent, discovered researchers at the University of South Carolina's Arnold School of Public Health. (If you weigh, say, 140 pounds, that works out to more than 2 pounds for every 30 tweets.) Researchers think Twitter keeps you accountable and gives real-time support.

11 **Kill the TV.** Keep in mind that trading in surfing on your laptop for lounging in front of the TV won't do your waistline any good: People who eat while glued to their flat screen down almost 300 more calories a day, according to a study from the University of Massachusetts. That would pretty much negate any calories burned during an exercise session! And it's now scientifically proven that reality bites: Food TV stokes your appetite . . . especially your sweet tooth, according to research in the journal *Appetite*. But some shows are worse for your diet than others. *Top Chef* is likelier to trigger an Oreo binge than say, *Worst Cooks in America* (we didn't feel that hungry either after seeing cohost Anne Burrell spit out her food in disgust!).

BIKINI DIET MEAL PLAN WEEK 1

Turn to the Month 1 Bikini Diet Meal Plan Cheat Sheet on page 22 for a quick overview on what to eat this week, or go to Chapter 14, page 163, for details on portion sizes and recipes. Remember to eliminate the 150 Flex Calories in this first Jump-Start Week to drop up to 3 pounds right off the bat.

If you're feeling really ravenous, remember the first rule for diet success: Eat for volume. Certain foods, such as veggies, are packed with fiber to help you feel satiated without being packed with calories that could derail your bikini body. To help tame your appetite as you're getting used to eating smaller portion sizes this week and skipping the daily Flex Calories, **feel free to add any of the following foods in the noted portions** to one of your daily snacks to help fill up your stomach without filling up on lots of extra calories (or any single serving of a fruit or veggie that has up to 45 calories and less than 1 gram of fat per serving):

1. Cucumber slices (only 10 calories per ½ cup)
2. Red bell pepper slices (only 10 calories per ½ cup)
3. Baby carrots (only 15 calories per 5 baby carrots)
4. Celery (only 10 calories per ½ cup)
5. Cauliflower (only 10 calories per ½ cup)
6. Broccoli (only 15 calories per ½ cup)
7. Air-popped popcorn (only 35 calories per cup)
8. Strawberries, sliced (only 30 calories per ½ cup)
9. Raspberries (only 40 calories per ½ cup)
10. Grapefruit (only 45 calories per ½ grapefruit)
11. Watermelon (only 45 calories per cup)
12. Peach (only 40 calories per medium peach)

HOT & HEALTHY WORKOUT WEEK 1

Your bikini body personal trainers Tracy Anderson and Barry and Joey of Barry's Bootcamp have crafted a fast-but-effective routine that makes sweating it out feel fun. Remember, the hardest part is getting started, but once you get into the groove, you'll feel totally energized.

Here's what to do this week:

◆ Morning Cardio Blast, 4 to 5 times this week, as soon as you wake up (See page 188.)
◆ Tracy Anderson's Tighten Up Your Butt toning routine, twice this week—but not on consecutive days! (See page 188.)
◆ Barry's Bootcamp Total-Body Strength Circuit, twice this week—but not on consecutive days! (See page 190.)
◆ Feel-Good Fitness day once this week (See page 194.)
◆ Rest and recover—2 days this week, but not on consecutive days!

HOW TO PLAN YOUR EARNED DAY

Hey, not everyone likes to stick to a set schedule all the time—and not everyone wants to follow a specific eating plan every single day of the week. This is where your earned day comes into play: It allows you some freedom as well as a little splurge to look forward to for eating healthy and fitting in fitness all week. The earned day helps you take control of your eating and builds in flexibility for your busy life. While it's not the green light to go crazy, it *is* a day to use all of the knowledge you have learned from the Bikini Diet for the week, while making your own food choices. (If the idea of going off the plan for a day freaks you out, instead choose one of your favorite days of meals.)

Here are some guidelines for planning your earned day.

◆ Have three meals and two snacks throughout the day paced out roughly every 3 to 4 hours! Remember, one

This week's 6-minute session from Tracy Anderson will tone and lift your backside at the same time to put some bam! in your booty. Sleek body bonus: The moves shown on page 188 work your core too, since your abs have to engage to help you balance. To max out the benefits, hold in your tummy as you do them and you'll flatten your belly ASAP.

The Total-Body Strength Circuit from Barry's Bootcamp: 20 Moves in 20 Minutes on page 190 will give get you sculpted all over by targeting each of your major bikini body parts while building muscle and igniting your metabolism. The month is divided into two phases: Phase 1 for the first 2 weeks calls for using 5- or 6-pound weights; phase 2 in weeks 3 and 4 helps you keep challenging your body by increasing the weights to 8 pounds. "If you're not feeling extremely fatigued, try upping the weights a little bit more no matter what phase you're in," says Joey Gonzalez, COO of Barry's Bootcamp. "You always want to feel the workout, but never want to sacrifice form."

Commit to following every aspect of the routine this first week to help you make fitting in fitness a habit and ensure your Bikini Diet success. Just think about how good you'll feel strutting on the beach with a tight, toned butt.

of those meals or snacks can veer off the Bikini Diet and be a real treat, such as hitting up your favorite pizza joint.

◆ Even when you're splurging on a decadent meal or dessert, remember the Bikini Diet Pledge: "I will pay attention to my appetite and pace my meals." When it comes to your daily meals, the goal is to simply stop when you are full (not when you have to unbutton your jeans!). Keep this in mind during your earned day and you won't go overboard.

◆ Sip mostly water!

◆ If you're going out to eat, research the restaurant options first to create your mealtime strategy for how to spend your calories. If you're eyeing up dessert, try sharing it with your friends and choose a lower-calorie meal to have enough wiggle room.

◆ If you're going to a friend's house, offer to bring along a healthy snack, like one of the Bikini Diet snacks, to share with all.

(UN)GUILTY PLEASURE: SLEEP YOUR WAY SKINNY

Did you know that you eat more and tend to crave high-fat, calorie-dense foods when you're tired? But will this knowledge motivate you to turn off *Chelsea Lately* to hit the sack? We're thinking probably not. (DVR, people!) Yet doing so will get you closer to your bikini body. Studies show that skimping on sleep leads to weight gain by decreasing leptin, a hormone that squelches appetite, and boosting ghrelin, another hormone that makes you hungry. Plus, lack of sleep can increase stress hormones, which might make you less efficient at metabolizing sugar and fats. Moreover, people who clock less than 7 hours of shut-eye a night are likelier to have more belly fat: Women snoozing less than 5 hours have waists that measure 5.4 centimeters larger than those who snooze for 7 to 8 hours, according to a study in *Obesity Reviews*.

Your feel-good goal this week is to clock at least 7 hours of sleep a night. An easy way to get your zzz's is through aromatherapy. (Don't roll your eyes—science backs it up!) When you inhale a calming scent like vanilla or lavender (a proven stress-hormone reducer), you reap the tension-melting, stress-calming benefits within minutes, says Laura Ann Conroy, a Bliss Spa educator. Try a room spray such as Molton Brown's Relaxing Yuan Zhi Ambiente. For maximum results, breathe in the aromas for a full 8 seconds, then breathe out for another 8 (repeat the series until you feel more chill). Last, set the mood for a great night's sleep by dimming your lights and turning off your TV, computer, and cell phone at least 20 minutes before bed—these electronic devices produce blue light waves, which have been found to interfere with sleep.

SUCCESS TRACKER:

Bikini Body Checklist Week 1

☐ I've starting watching my serving sizes and tried the Cosmo Bikini Diet tricks for keeping portions in check.

☐ I've followed the Meal Plan for the Jump-Start Week.

☐ I've followed the secrets for dieting success, like looking up nutrition information online before eating at a restaurant.

☐ I've made an energizing playlist to help keep me motivated during my workouts.

☐ I've followed the Hot & Healthy Workout plan.

☐ I've clocked (or at least tried to clock) seven hours of sleep a night.

Week 1 Measurements

Weight_____

Waist_____

Chest_____

Hips_____

This week I feel _____

_____

_____

_____

_____

_____

_____

_____

_____

_____

CHAPTER TWO

EAT BREAKFAST TO SLIM DOWN

WEEK #2

THE LOWDOWN Good news! This week we're giving you more new and delicious breakfasts to choose from. That's because the old saying is true: Breakfast really is the most important meal of the day.

When compared to breakfast eaters, people who skip breakfast actually down 40 percent more sweets; 55 percent more soft drinks; 45 percent fewer vegetables, and 30 percent less fruit. So eat up! Mornings just got a whole lot more delicious.

We'll also show you that nutritious eating doesn't have to be expensive and which healthy breakfast staples will fatten your wallet while slimming your waistline. To keep you motivated to stick to the Cosmo Bikini Diet meal plans and Hot & Healthy Workouts all week long, we'll provide some celeb bikini-bod love and other inspiring tricks to help you reach your goals.

Seriously, you won't even feel like you're on a diet, because we'll also tell you why planning a food splurge and pampering yourself with feel-good moments every single day will help you shed pounds.

WHY EATING BREAKFAST MAKES YOU SKINNY

Still subsisting on nothing but coffee before noon? Sure, eating may not be your utmost concern when trying to beat your boss into the office, but contrary to the common belief that skipping breakfast saves you calories, studies show that people who didn't eat a morning meal made worse food choices and actually ate more calories later on. That's because having brekkie may curb hunger so you don't overeat at lunch and helps you make healthier food choices for the rest of the day to better keep pounds at bay. In fact, almost 80 percent of people who lost 30 pounds or more and kept it off eat breakfast, according to the National Weight Control Registry.

Eating first thing in the a.m. also fuels your metabolism for the rest of the day. While you want to hold off on eating until right after your 15 minutes of daily cardio (which should be done as soon as you wake up), waiting more than an hour and a half or so to have breakfast only starts you off low on energy and in a funk. Your brain runs on glucose, which dips if you haven't eaten all night, making you feel foggy, less equipped to deal with stress, and more likely to cave when cravings strike. **Make sure that your breakfast is built around protein and healthy fats with some high-quality, low-sugar carbohydrates thrown in the mix.** (And that's exactly the kind of breakfasts we've designed for you.) Research shows protein stimulates metabolism and fat keeps you feeling fuller longer to help maintain a healthy weight. Mixing in carbohydrates gives you a quick energy boost so you can tackle your day.

MOVE IN THE MORNING, EAT LESS

The secret to rock-hard willpower (and abs)? Working out in the a.m. Scientists at Brigham Young University measured the neural activity of women who exercised in the morning versus women who didn't, and it turns out those who got their butts in gear early were less responsive to images of food. In other words, they weren't as tempted by food. So think of your 15-minute morning cardio interval as defense against your coworker's latest Pinterest-inspired cookie/cake/calorie bomb.

HEALTHY BUDGET BREAKFAST STAPLES

Eating in the a.m. is not only good for your waistline...it's also a cheap way to pack in a lot of your day's nutrients. That's because many go-to breakfast ingredients are both high in nutrients and budget friendly. Maybe you think you can't afford to eat healthy all the time, but it's pretty much a myth that nutritious food costs more than junk food: When families switched to healthier diets and lost weight, the money they spent on their food budget dropped, while their meals packed more protein and nutrients, according to a study in the *Journal of the American Dietetic Association*.

CELEB BIKINI BODY LOVE

These stars have sexy, healthy bikini bodies. Here's why we love them.

Beyoncé Rather than get down on herself for gaining a few pounds, the famously curvy singer wrote the song "Bootylicious" to help other women channel their inner sexiness—regardless of whether or not you can squeeze into your skinny jeans.

Kelly Clarkson

Though she dropped 18 pounds from downsizing her portions and spending more time biking in the great outdoors, she's not obsessed with being skinny.

Rather, her focus is on feeling good and being a badass singer. "I want to be a healthy individual—which I always have been," she told Cosmo.

Selena Gomez

Sure, there's lots of pressure on young singers and actresses to have the perfect bod (wouldn't *you* freak out if the paparazzi was taking pictures of you on the beach that you knew would make front page tabloid news?). Talk about pressure. Selena said it's exhausting, so she'd rather focus on embracing what God gave her. She's said, "I feel that there's a point in everybody's life where

they think that they're not perfect and they look in the mirror and see what could be better. And one of my best friends told me to get up every morning and try to say to yourself, 'I am beautiful,' every single morning. And that helped a lot."

Vanessa Hudgens

Though she's gotten some flack from the press for filling out a bit since her *High School Musical* days, Vanessa told *Access Hollywood*, "My body is my body. . . I love myself and I think you've got to be proud of the body you have and own it. . . "

For example, running into your local deli for a greasy sausage, egg, and cheese sandwich on a roll may cost $5. Scramble two eggs in heart-healthy olive oil at home and serve on a slice of whole-grain toast, and you'll be down less than $1. (Yearly savings: $1,460, or the cost of a beach vacation!) And a yogurt parfait may run about $3.50 when eating out, but making your own with higher-protein Greek yogurt, half a sliced banana, and a handful of crunchy cereal would cost you about $1.50 per serving. (Yearly savings: $730)

So while you may be tempted to grab a fast-food breakfast on the go thinking that you're eating light while saving calories and money, know that that grande white

Jennifer Lawrence

When *The Hunger Games* starlet faced critics who said she was too fat for the role of Katniss Everdeen, rather than swearing off carbs and going on a liquid diet, she stood up and said that she was proud that she didn't fit the stereotypical stick-thin Hollywood mold because her body is healthy and normal. Then she went on to score a lead role—and an Oscar for Best Actress—as sexy Tiffany in the hit film *Silver Linings Playbook*. In your face, haters!

Leighton Meester

The svelte actress does strength-training workouts outdoors. She also incorporates the Cosmo Bikini Diet philosophy of making time for pleasure, relaxation, and de-stressing by taking 5 minutes to meditate before each sweat session.

Pink The muscular pop star rocks the stage with confidence. And for her, beauty is more than skin deep. "Beautiful has never been my goal. Joy is my goal—to feel healthy and strong and powerful and useful and engaged and intelligent and in love," she says.

Rihanna She looks white-hot in a bikini, but she sticks to a healthy lifestyle rather than yo-yo diets to keep her toned bod. She squeezes in at least three workouts a week while she's on the road, and is also rumored to follow celebrity trainer Harley Pasternak's diet advice of eating five meals a day that all have the healthy combo of protein, fiber, quality carbs, and fats. That's a surefire recipe for holding on to her bikini bod during any season.

Jordin Sparks

The youngest winner of *American Idol* lost 30 pounds by adopting a healthier lifestyle instead of going on a deprivation diet. She's proof that making small, healthy changes is the best way to get lean and to keep the weight off for good!

chocolate mocha with whipped cream packs 470 calories and 18 grams of fat alone—and could cost you about $4, depending on where you live. (Brewing up your own cup at home and adding a splash of milk will cost you only about 25 cents!) And that high calorie count for just one drink is *before* you throw in a nutrient-light blueberry muffin (460 calories, 15 grams of fat) or a plain old bagel with cream cheese (460 calories, 16 grams of fat). Instead, stock your kitchen with these breakfast staples that are low in cost but high in nutrition.

You'll find these breakfast staples in this week's meal plan. Remember: You can always choose to eat any one of the suggested breakfasts on any day you like.

EGGS (17 CENTS EACH)

Having an egg first thing in the a.m. fills you up with 6 grams of protein to help control your appetite until lunch. Take full advantage of the nutritional benefits by eating the yolk, too: It's packed with powerhouse nutrients such as choline, which is important for brainpower and mood.

BUILD A BETTER BOWL OF OATMEAL

If you don't have time to make slow-cooked oats (see page 81), trick out your plain ol' packet of instant with these tasty and nutritious a.m. add-ons.

Honey Crunch
Add a teaspoon of honey, 1 tablespoon walnuts, and ¼ teaspoon cinnamon to cooked oatmeal.

Peanut Butter Banana
Stir 1 teaspoon natural peanut butter into cooked oatmeal, and top with ½ cup sliced bananas.

Tomato & Cheese
Top cooked oatmeal with ¼ cup shredded Cheddar cheese (reduced fat or 2% light), 1 tablespoon diced red onion, and ¼ cup diced tomato.

Tropical Delight
Top cooked oatmeal with ¼ cup diced pineapple, ¼ cup diced mango, 1 tablespoon shredded coconut, and a splash (⅛ cup or less) low-fat milk or almond milk.

◆ **Make it a meal:** Have an egg scrambled in a teaspoon of heart-healthy olive oil on half of a whole wheat English muffin or a slice of whole-grain toast for filling fiber and a healthy carb-protein-fat combo.

COFFEE (18 CENTS A CUP)

Your morning cup of joe is a good source of flavonoids, a disease-fighting antioxidant. More good news for all of you caffeine addicts: Studies show that caffeine (in moderation) can have surprising health benefits, such as boosting your exercise and mental performance, stabilizing blood sugars, and even warding off Alzheimer's later in life.
◆ **Make it a meal:** Add calcium to your coffee by having a skim latte. Throw a hard-boiled egg and a piece of fruit into a bag and you're good to go.

PEANUT BUTTER (18 CENTS PER SERVING)

Just 1 tablespoon has 4 grams of protein, 8 grams of fat, a few grams of fiber, and only 4 grams of carbs. Plus, it's packed with polyunsaturated fatty acids that help lower cholesterol while keeping you feeling full longer to control appetite.
◆ **Make it a meal:** Top a whole-grain English muffin with 2 teaspoons peanut butter, ½ sliced banana, and a drizzle of honey for a mix of healthy fats, fiber, and protein.

OLD-FASHIONED ROLLED OATS (22 CENTS A SERVING)

Processed cereals can be a sneaky source of sugar, so it's best to opt for no-sugar-added whole grains in the a.m. Oats are a great choice because they've also been shown to lower bad cholesterol.
◆ **Make it a meal:** Mix a cup each rolled oats and fat-free milk with a teaspoon each almonds and dried fruit. Microwave for 4 minutes, then let sit another minute so the oats soak up the liquid.

GREEK YOGURT (ABOUT $1.10 PER 6-OUNCE CONTAINER)

Though Greek yogurt may have a slightly higher price tag than the regular kind, you'll get more nutrition for your money: The Greek kind has about 16 grams of protein compared to about 7 grams in the regular stuff. Buy it plain to cut down on sugar and cost. Be sure to check the label for gut-protecting bacteria *L. acidophilus* and *B. bifidum*, and the "Live and Active Cultures" seal.
◆ **Make it a meal:** Flavor plain Greek yogurt with honey, cinnamon, and sliced bananas for a sweet start to your day. You'll notice that smaller portions of Greek yogurt may also be listed as a snack idea throughout the monthly meal plans. The satiating carb-protein-fat combos that we've built the breakfasts around also make satisfying snacks in slightly smaller portion sizes.

BANANAS (31 CENTS PER SERVING)

Bananas are both cheap and portable. Snack on a banana for a jolt before Zumba or a Spinning class; it'll score you more endurance than downing a sports drink, research shows. Why? Bananas have a healthier blend of natural sugars plus higher potassium levels, a crucial mineral that helps you stay hydrated.

◆ **Make it a meal:** Dip a small banana in 1 tablespoon peanut butter sprinkled with cinnamon. Bonus: Cinnamon adds flavor without adding calories, and also helps control spikes in blood sugar.

WHOLE WHEAT BREAD (12 CENTS PER 1-SLICE SERVING)

Breads made with whole grains keep your blood sugar levels from spiking so you don't get a midmorning energy crash like you would when eating the white kind, because they're less processed and so take longer to digest. Some breads may claim to be whole wheat or whole grain even if they've been highly processed, so first check the ingredient list to make sure the words *whole grain* or *whole wheat* are first, and then look at the nutrition label to ensure there's at least 2 to 3 grams of fiber per serving.

◆ **Make it a meal:** Dunk whole wheat bread in a mixture of eggs and cinnamon and brown in a pan for healthy French toast. Top with berries, sliced apples, bananas, or no-sugar-added jam instead of syrup to cut down on sugar and calories.

SPINACH ($1.30 PER SERVING)

Here's another reason to eat your greens: Spinach is high in iron, which helps transport oxygen throughout your body to keep you from feeling sluggish and help boost your workouts. Drizzle with lemon juice, because vitamin C–rich foods make it easier for your body to absorb iron.

◆ **Make it a meal:** Add a side of steamed spinach to your eggs to get an extra 6 milligrams of iron. Women need 18 milligrams a day, so you'll have reached one-third of your daily intake at breakfast.

LOW-FAT MILK (23 CENTS A CUP)

Besides being a great source of bone-strengthening calcium, milk has vitamin B, potassium, and vitamin D. It's also high in leucine, an amino acid needed for muscle growth. One study found exercisers who drank milk lost 40 percent more fat and gained 63 percent more muscle compared to those having a soy beverage, reports the *American Journal of Clinical Nutrition.*

◆ **Make it a meal:** Add milk to your rolled oats instead of water. It'll taste creamier and keep you feeling satisfied longer because of the extra protein.

BIKINI DIET MEAL PLAN WEEK 2

Turn to the Month 1 Bikini Diet Meal Plan Cheat Sheet on page 22 for a quick overview of what to eat this week, or go to Chapter 14, page 163, for details on portion sizes and recipes. Since this chapter is all about breakfast, notice which a.m. food combos give you the most energy and keep you feeling satisfied until lunchtime rolls around. As you get deeper into the Cosmo Bikini Diet, you can stick to the breakfast foods that give you the right amount of energy to get through your busy mornings. Here are some make-ahead grab-and-go breakfast ideas that save time so you can still beat your boss into the office. Swap these for the breakfasts in the meal plan if you need to get going in a hurry.

◆ Hard-boiling protein-packed eggs makes them portable. Store them in a to-go container, then throw two in a bag with a piece of fruit, such as a banana.
◆ Mix berry smoothies to store in the fridge by blending 1 cup fat-free milk, 3 ice cubes, 2 tablespoons flaxseed, and 1 ¼ cups frozen strawberries or blackberries.
◆ Put together a portable breakfast pack that includes a plastic bowl and spoon with baggies portioned out with ¾ cup shredded wheat (or other high-fiber cereal) and a teaspoon each of walnuts and raisins. Grab a small carton of fat-free milk and you're good to go.
◆ Make a batch of steel-cut oats on the weekends and divide it into portion-controlled Tupperware packs. Then grab the container and heat in the microwave. Stir in sliced apples, cinnamon, and a drizzle of maple syrup for taste.
◆ Take a container of Greek yogurt (we love Chobani's pomegranate flavor), and pair it with a baggie of 10 to 12 salted almonds for added healthy fat and protein.

MY BIKINI BODY SLIMSPIRATION

Being able to envision the bikini body you want makes it easier to make the right daily choices—such as choosing a healthy snack or fitting in your 15 minutes of cardio first thing in the morning—that will get you closer to your goal. Flip through mags such as Cosmo to find pictures of women's bodies that are strong, healthy, and rock a bikini to provide visual inspiration to stick to the plan. Snap photos of them with your phone so you'll always have a photo gallery on hand for inspiration—or try pinning your fave bikini body celebs to your Pinterest board. Just be sure you're choosing bodies that are realistic for your particular type to keep from getting discouraged. Like if you're 5'1" and curvy like Salma Hayek, it's probably not a good idea to create a collage of lanky, 5'11" body types like Taylor Swift.

Also, go to Cosmo's Pinterest page (pinterest.com/cosmopolitan) that features rocking bikini bods. Post pictures of women who inspire you to get in shape.

HOT & HEALTHY WORKOUT WEEK 2

You're already on week 2 of the Cosmo Bikini Diet! While you may be feeling a burst of energy on some days during your workouts, don't be discouraged if you find yourself dragging on others. Remember, it takes time to adapt to a new, healthy lifestyle! Stick it out this week and we guarantee that your new fitness routine will not only get easier, but you'll also start to feel stronger. Look to your Bikini Body Slimspiration images of women with strong, sexy bods as motivation to fit in all of your workouts this week.

You can stick to using 5- or 6-pound weights this week for the Total-Body Strength Circuit from Barry's Bootcamp—but up your weights if the routine already feels too easy! And this week's quick toning moves from Tracy Anderson also work multiple body parts at once to get you leaner all over. By exercising several trouble zones simultaneously, you'll torch extra calories, since more muscles are engaged.

Here's what to do this week:

◆ Morning Cardio Blast, 4 to 5 times this week, as soon as you wake up (See page 195.)
◆ Tracy Anderson's Tone Up Three Times Faster toning routine, twice this week—but not on consecutive days! (See page 196.)
◆ Barry's Bootcamp Total-Body Strength Circuit, twice this week—but not on consecutive days! (See page 195.)
◆ Feel-Good Fitness day once this week (See page 197.)
◆ Rest and recover—2 days this week, but not on consecutive days!

(UN)GUILTY PLEASURE: PLAN A SPLURGE

If you're depriving yourself of your fave food, you're likely to eat more of other foods and do more bikini body damage than if you'd just allowed yourself a small portion of what you were lusting after in the first place. Sometimes a low-fat cheese stick just won't ease your pizza craving, and dried fruit simply can't replace peach cobbler. Ditching the diet mentality and allowing yourself small portions of decadent foods can help prevent cravings altogether. You can scoop half a cup of ice cream into a Tupperware container and store it in your freezer, if you know that's what you'll reach for at 8 p.m. That way, you can eat what you really want without consuming a lot of extra calories. Try anticipating your splurges at the beginning of the day. Since you'll know it's coming, it will be so much easier to keep portions in check.

SUCCESS TRACKER:

Bikini Body Checklist Week 2

☐ I've eaten a healthy breakfast every day this week and noted which food combos best kept me going 'til lunch.

☐ I've stocked my kitchen with healthy-budget breakfast staples.

☐ I've created my Bikini Body Slimspiration Pinterest board or photo gallery on my cell and look at it daily as a reminder to stick to my exercise and meal-plan goals.

☐ I've followed the Hot & Healthy Workout plan.

☐ I've planned a splurge to allow myself something delicious while keeping cravings in check.

Week 2 Measurements

Weight _____

Waist _____

Chest _____

Hips _____

This week I feel _____

_____

_____

_____

_____

_____

_____

_____

_____

_____

_____

_____

CHAPTER THREE

FUEL UP YOUR EXERCISE

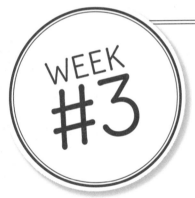

THE LOWDOWN To max out the slimming and toning benefits of your workout, it's crucial to start with a foundation of healthy eating that delivers the nutrients your body needs to perform at its best. We've already taken care of "what to eat?" with the weekly meal plans. Also important is knowing *when* you should eat so you get the most out of your exercise routine.

This chapter includes:
◆ Which types of foods best fuel your workouts and exactly when to eat them to reap the biggest benefits
◆ The top weight-loss myths that may be holding you back from getting the body you've always dreamed about
◆ Whether or not you should weigh in daily
◆ Small tricks for getting bigger workout results
◆ How having an orgasm might help you lose weight

TIMING MEALS AROUND EXERCISE

If you're not eating the right nutrients at the right times, your sweat sessions might send your appetite into overdrive. And who wants to spend time at the gym only to see it wasted because you ended up eating *more* calories than you burned? Follow these tips to eat smarter before and after exercise to help control appetite, supply the nutrients your body needs for peak performance, speed up muscle recovery, and get toned faster.

Rather than viewing your pre- and postworkout snacks as calories going in, think about it more as a way to keep your blood sugar levels steady so you can work out harder and recover faster. "It's like giving fuel to your car before a road trip. When you focus on eating nutrient-dense foods at the proper pre- and postworkout times, you'll maximize your training session and control appetite so you ultimately lose more weight—despite eating some extra calories in order to sustain yourself," says Mike Dolce, designer of UFC FIT (ufcfit.com) and creator of *The Dolce Diet*. Since you get two snacks a day, you can try timing your snacks around your exercise sessions to get the best sculpting results.

What to eat before exercise: It's key to do your 15-minute morning cardio intervals on an empty stomach to put your bod into optimal fat-burning mode for the rest of the day. This is the only time in the program you should *not* eat before exercise. But don't skip a preworkout snack when it comes to lifting weights or doing longer sweat sessions (this is especially important when you increase the length of your Total-Body Strength Circuit from Barry's Bootcamp sessions in month 3). Lifting weights on an empty stomach makes you more likely to burn muscle—which ultimately slows metabolism—since your muscles won't have any glycogen or sugar supplies from food to use as a fuel source.

"Eat a preworkout snack anywhere from 45 to 90 minutes before your training session so you can push yourself harder to achieve the best results," says Dolce. Just a reminder: This snack would spend your Flex Calories for the day or take the place of another Bikini Diet snack. Try these tasty and portable 150-calorie preworkout snacks with 16 ounces of water to fuel your workout. Each includes carbs, some protein, and some fat.

- an apple with a handful (½ ounce) of almonds (11 almonds)
- a few ounces raisins with a handful of sunflower seeds
- a small banana mashed and topped with 1 tablespoon chopped walnuts and 1 teaspoon honey
- 5 whole wheat crackers topped with a ¾-ounce mini Babybel cheese (or other ¾-ounce cheese that's 70 calories)
- 6 honey wheat pretzel sticks with 2 teaspoons peanut butter
- ¼ cup dried cranberries with 5 almonds
- 6 ounces fat-free or low-fat Greek yogurt

- ½ cup brown rice cereal topped with ¼ cup low-fat milk and ½ cup of sliced bananas
- 5 whole wheat crackers topped with 2 tablespoons hummus

What to have during exercise: No need to eat during the Cosmo Bikini Diet workouts, but just be sure to drink 4 to 6 ounces of water every 15 to 20 minutes of exercise to keep hydrated while you're sweating it out.

What to eat after exercise: You might tend to skip a snack after working out because you don't want to consume calories that you just burned. However, refueling your body after a workout is a must to help refuel your tired muscles. Ideally, you'd plan to have one of your Bikini Diet snacks or use your Flex Calories for the day within 30 minutes of working out, although there's a 2-hour window postexercise where your muscles are like a sponge, waiting for fuel (aka food) to repair and replenish those muscles to get ready for your next workout.

LIQUID ENERGY

These unexpected beverages deliver big-time workout boosts.

Try Beet Juice . . .
when training for a 5K
Sip beet juice for a few days before your event and you may finish faster. Nitrate compounds are thought to improve blood flow to muscles.

Try Coffee . . .
before strength or cardio
Caffeine delays how quickly you have to use glycogen for energy, so you can spin/lift/Zumba/do your fave workout even longer.

Try Chocolate Milk . . .
after strength or cardio
The combo of carbs and protein speedily repairs (normal) postworkout microtears, reducing soreness. The magic window: within 30 minutes of your session.

Try Nonalcoholic Beer . . .
after a half marathon
Endurance events can weaken your immunity, but anti-inflammatory compounds in nonalcoholic beer may thwart the effect.

When to have your postexercise meal: "If you're doing a higher-intensity workout that involves weights or strength training, be sure to eat a meal within 90 minutes of exercise to keep your metabolism revved and aid in muscle repair," says Dolce. So whether you're doing your lifting sessions before lunch or dinner, don't let hours go by before you sit down for a balanced meal. The Cosmo Bikini Diet meal plan includes the ideal combo of the protein, high-quality carbs, and healthy fats that your body needs to optimize your exercise sessions.

TOP 10 WEIGHT-LOSS MYTHS—BUSTED!

When it comes to shaping up, some common beliefs may be holding you back from attaining your goals. "Many diets call for deprivation, but weight-loss plans must be sustainable as well as enjoyable in order to change your body—and your life—for good," says Dolce. Check out the all-time biggest diet myths and how to overcome them so you can get the body you've always wanted.

1 **I have to count calories in order to lose weight.** "It's absolutely wrong," says Dolce. "I know from training elite athletes that the *quality* of calories matters much more than the *quantity*." Aim to eat nutrient-dense foods instead of focusing on eating only low-calorie foods, because it's what's inside those calories that really counts. "Eating only 100-calorie packs of crackers or cookies as opposed to having, say, a handful of blueberries and walnuts, means you're missing vital nutrients such as amino acids needed to repair muscles after your workout," says Dolce. "Plus, processed carbs won't stabilize your blood sugar levels, so you won't feel as good after eating them."

2 **Lifting weights will make me bulky.** Lifting weights won't turn you into a man—it'll leave you looking more toned. And a strong, shapely body *never* looks bad. "You don't necessarily have to lose weight in order to look better, you just need to build muscle to lift and tighten," says Dolce. "Even gaining one pound of muscle from lifting will reduce your body fat percentage and change the shape of your body." While using dumbbells and resistance bands can definitely maximize your results, simply using your own body weight by doing 5 minutes of squats every morning will help lift your butt. Be sure to keep this in mind if the scale seems to get stuck, because you could actually be gaining muscle mass and losing inches, making your clothes fit better, yet the number on the scale reads the same.

3 **Protein powders and diet pills can help me slim down faster.** Protein powders may play a role for some athletes, although when it comes to slimming down, there's no magic pill that will make you lose weight. "If those pills worked, we'd all be skinny," says Dolce. "Instead, diet pills are selling better than ever and we're only getting

fatter than ever as a nation." Powders, potions, and pills sound like a quick fix, but even if they worked they wouldn't last, because you can't live off them forever. Sure, adopting a healthy eating and exercise routine takes time, but you'll be able to hold on to the results once you've made those lifestyle changes. "Your progress becomes exponential because those small, little victories add up over time," says Dolce. "Before you know it, you'll be wearing that string bikini that you've always dreamed about and feeling great in it."

4 **Cardio is the best way to burn body fat.** "Doing excessive cardio actually breaks down muscle tissue to boost body fat storage. This is how you see those people who are skinny fat," says Dolce. "They fit into smaller sizes but look bad naked. That's not what we want. We want to be tight and toned." Strength training increases muscle mass for a thermogenic effect, so you burn more calories even while sitting still rather than hold on to body fat, and you look more toned overall. "When I say cardio, I'm talking about aerobic exercise like spending an hour on the treadmill and not the anaerobic kind such as 15 minutes of high-intensity intervals," says Dolce. "You'd be better off spending an hour relaxing in a warm bath than killing yourself on a treadmill, since de-stressing is another important secret to getting your best body."

SHOULD YOU WEIGH IN EVERY DAY?

YES! according to J. Graham Thomas, PhD, coinvestigator at the National Weight Control Registry at Brown University, a program that tracks successful dieters.

"Stepping on a scale once a day will help prevent extra pounds from creeping up on you. It's difficult to keep tabs on everything you consume, and having a number to go on is the only reliable way to know where you stand. Otherwise, you may not notice you've gained weight until it's more than a few pounds and much harder to get rid of.

"In addition to being a tracking tool, the scale is a psychological reminder that measured eating pays off. For the rest of the day, you'll feel more motivated to eat and drink in moderation. It may sound scary to face the music on a daily basis, but it'll reinforce your willpower when you're tempted to overindulge."

5 **Carbohydrates pack on the pounds.** Carbs are essential for all of our body functions. In fact, carbs break down into glucose, which is the number-one preferred source of fuel for the brain, plus carbs fuel muscles with the energy to exercise. "The key is to eat nutrient-dense carbs rather than the processed kind," says Dolce (see page 87). "So I'm not talking about eating a bagel for breakfast, but instead having slow-cooked rolled oats mixed with flaxseeds and sliced apple."

6 **No pain, no gain.** "The idea that you have to kill yourself at the gym in order to see results is ridiculous, outdated, and old-school," says Dolce. "It's about bringing *intelligent intensity* to your workout, where you push yourself to the point of progress and then go home to rest to let your body repair." Pushing yourself too hard to the point where you can't get out of bed the next day not only makes exercise feel like torture, but it also makes you less likely to stick with it.

7 **I need cheat meals to help me stay on track.** "I don't believe in cheat meals at all, because I think they're an excuse for people to be lazy," says Dolce. "Do you cheat on your partner? Do you cheat on a test? Why would you want to

NO! according to Brian Wansink, PhD, director of the Cornell University Food and Brand Lab and author of *Mindless Eating: Why We Eat More Than We Think*. "A daily weigh-in can be discouraging and counterproductive. It's frustrating to detect the normal, day-to-day variations in your weight, which can go up 3 to 4 pounds depending on when you ate your last meal and where you are in your cycle. Seeing what's likely a temporary uptick might make you throw in the towel, thinking you're already too far gone and there's no point in watching your intake. Also, obsessing over your weight can create a negative cycle in which you deprive yourself, then binge, so you wind up eating more.

"As long as you keep exercising, a few rich meals won't have a noticeable impact on your size. Use your jeans as a gauge; they're a less stressful way to monitor your shape than fretting over a number," Wansink says.

cheat on your health and your body? Instead, try rewarding yourself with *earned* meals after you've met a specific goal." Go ahead and enjoy that slice of pizza once you've dropped a dress size, or treat yourself to a banana split if you've succeeded in increasing your weights during your lifting routine. The next day, get right back into your healthy-eating regimen until you can reward yourself again for your next mission accomplished.

8 I have to start out doing "girl" push-ups. "There's no such thing as "girl" CEOs—you're either CEO or you're not," says Dolce. "Likewise, there is no such thing as "girl" push-ups—there are only modifications for beginner, immediate, and advanced. I've seen plenty of girls who can do better push-ups than some of the guys."

Rather than automatically taking the easy route, constantly push yourself to the next level for better results. Maybe you can do 10 regular push-ups before you have to put your knees on the floor—or maybe you can only do five. "As long as you understand your abilities in this moment, then you can accurately assess what you need to do and how you need to move forward," says Dolce. "You have to respect your current ability in order to make the fastest progress."

9 Fat-spot reduction is key. "No matter how many crunches we do, we're not going to melt away belly fat," says Dolce. "The only thing that reduces fat in specific spots on our body is a 24-hour-a-day lifestyle change, and not spending an hour in the gym." So in order to zap cellulite and see your new firmer, more shapely butt, you have to adopt an overall healthy routine. That means doing your 15 minutes of morning intervals, getting enough rest, and taking time for yourself to, say, mentally unplug and listen to your favorite playlist. Once you've made these healthy changes, the quick body-part-specific toning sessions in the Hot & Healthy Workouts will become even more effective as your bikini body takes shape.

"Most people think a healthy lifestyle has to be work, but it's something you should embrace because it's fulfilling and makes you happier," say Dolce. "Living a life that nourishes your body and spirit is empowering. You don't have to be a skinny-minny model, you just have to look good for you."

10 I need a gym membership to see results. Forget going all the way to the gym and back to fit in an effective workout (unless you want to!): All you need is a 6-by-6-foot space. "That's literally a body's length in front of your TV or bed or in your hotel room," says Dolce. "That's enough space to do 15 to 45 minutes of intervals or resistance moves, such as squats and push-ups. Or you can simply walk out of your front door and do sprint repeats to your mailbox and back for 20 minutes. No gym required!"

BIKINI DIET MEAL PLAN WEEK 3

Turn to the Month 1 Bikini Diet Meal Plan Cheat Sheet on page 22 for a quick overview on what to eat this week, or go to Chapter 14, page 163, for details on portion sizes and recipes. Also on the days you have longer workouts, try swapping in some of the pre- and postworkout snacks suggested on page 49 in place of the snacks listed in the month 1 meal plan.

SIMPLE TRICKS TO GET LEANER IN NO TIME

These moves from Tracy Anderson will help you get more out of your workout, so you'll tone up even faster.

Pump up your playlist. Listening to fast-paced music can help you exercise longer. A study found that when participants listened to rock or pop, they had 15 percent more endurance than those who worked out tune free.

Mix it up. Changing your routine makes you more likely to hit the gym, according to research. So alternate between the elliptical and Spinning class, for example.

Work out next to the gym rat. Hop onto a treadmill next to a person who's running fast, or stand beside the woman in a body-pump exercise class who's a pro. A recent study proved that just being near someone who's giving it her all will cause you to break more of a sweat too.

Vary your tempo. Don't underestimate the fat-burning power of your 15 minutes of morning-cardio sessions! Instead of maintaining a steady pace during cardio, go superquick for short spurts of time (for example, walk for 3 minutes, then sprint for 1 minute, for a total of 15 to 30 minutes). One study found that female cyclists who alternated between pedaling fast and going easy burned three times more fat than women who cycled at a fixed speed did.

HOT & HEALTHY WORKOUT WEEK 3

Now that you've got 2 solid weeks behind you, keep challenging your body for optimum results. This week, you'll up your weights to 8 pounds for the Total-Body Strength Circuit from Barry's Bootcamp. And Tracy Anderson's Slim Your Waist toning routine gets you a toned, flat tummy—incredibly fast. As you get stronger, hold the plank and bridge poses for a bit longer—even just a second or two—to tighten your midsection more quickly.

Here's what to do this week:

◆ Morning Cardio Blast, 4 to 5 times this week, as soon as you wake up (See page 198.)
◆ Tracy Anderson's Slim Your Waist toning routine, twice this week—but not on consecutive days! (See page 199.)
◆ Barry's Bootcamp Total-Body Strength Circuit, twice this week—but not on consecutive days! (See page 198.)
◆ Feel-Good Fitness day once this week (See page 200.)
◆ Rest and recover—2 days this week, but not on consecutive days!

(UN)GUILTY PLEASURE: HOW SEX CAN MAKE YOU SKINNIER

A growing body of research suggests that not only do refined carbs—like pasta, cake, croissants, and white rice—cause us to gain weight (by driving the body to store excess sugar as fat), but for some people, they're also addictive. "Processed carbs and simple sugars are devoid of nutrients, fat, fiber, and protein—all the things that take a while to digest and provide lasting satiety," says Andrew Lawson, MD, coauthor of *Clean Cuisine*. "They give you a brief feel-good rush, and when it's over, you want more."

Dr. Mehmet Oz has floated a new theory that sex can curb a carb craving. The (admittedly not very scientific) idea is this: The rush you get from refined carbs comes when they trigger the release of the feel-good hormone serotonin in your brain. But sexual arousal emits a powerful happiness hormone of its own: oxytocin. So it follows from Dr. Oz's theory that when you crave the comfort of some cheesecake, why not reach for a condom instead? "Theoretically, this could work," agrees Dr. Lawson, albeit cautiously.

Whether or not the theory of sex as a weight-loss strategy can be proven, having a big O is a guaranteed feel-good way to distract yourself from tearing into that box of cookies that's calling your name. Plus, regular sex sessions tune you in to your body, so you may pay more attention to hunger and fullness cues. At the very least, spending an hour getting it on burns about 100 calories. So take time out for a little sexual healing this week—solo or with a partner—and your bikini body will thank you.

SUCCESS TRACKER:

Bikini Body Checklist Week 3

- ☐ I've eaten a small snack that includes a healthy combo of carbs, fat, and protein before my longer workout sessions.
- ☐ I've eaten a protein-packed snack within 30 minutes of finishing exercise.
- ☐ I've changed my mind-set to overcome the most common weight-loss myths.
- ☐ I've followed the Bikini Diet meal plan.
- ☐ I've followed the Hot & Healthy Workout plan.
- ☐ I've taken time out to have a big O to get more in tune with my body.

Week 3 Measurements

Weight_____

Waist_____

Chest_____

Hips_____

This week I feel _____

_____
_____
_____
_____
_____
_____
_____
_____
_____
_____
_____
_____

CHAPTER FOUR

GET A HANDLE ON EMOTIONAL EATING

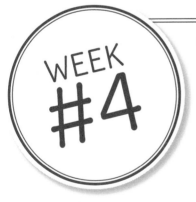

WEEK
#4

THE LOWDOWN While both eating right and exercising are essential for getting your strongest, sexiest shape, so is controlling what goes on inside your head. That's because achieving your most beautiful figure may be more about changing your mind-set and ditching the emotional clutter than about merely counting calories or kicking butt at the gym.

Think about it: Have you ever crashed on the couch after a tough day at work or a fight with your BF, distracting yourself with a bottle of wine and a pint of ice cream (or whatever your go-to comfort food may be)? While occasionally feeding your face to soothe yourself won't make you fat, living on overdrive with no time to unwind except for quick fixes like comfort food—as opposed to facing your feelings—will definitely take its toll on your mind *and* your body.

This week we'll help you better recognize your emotional-eating triggers and give you the tools you need to halt emotional eating for good. You'll also learn celebrity trainer secrets for getting lean thighs without lunges and how eating away from your desk can help you nosh less.

WHAT ARE YOU HUNGRY FOR?

It's 3 p.m., and suddenly you *have* to have a candy bar, or you can't stop thinking about those chips in the company snack room. You ate lunch, so why can't you get sweet or salty snacks off your mind? There are many reasons why you experience cravings. "Sometimes it's emotional and you reach for foods that you love for comfort," says Molly Morgan, RD, author of *The Skinny Rules*. "Other times, it may be that you're tired, which triggers the release of hormones linked to hunger." Sometimes you simply haven't eaten enough calories and you really *do* need to nosh for energy.

So how can you tell if your eating is triggered by emotions or real hunger? "If you're having cravings at the same time every day, such as at 3 p.m., it could be because you're not getting what your body needs earlier in the day, such as protein. You might try eating something different for breakfast or lunch to see if, say, adding more protein or fiber helps you feel full for longer. On the other hand, if your cravings start each night right after you've had a decent-size dinner, it's probably more emotional, such as stress or boredom," says Morgan.

If you're starting to recognize that you're eating emotionally rather than munching out of true hunger, it's vital to get to the root cause of *why* you sometimes binge. "Most people think they overeat because they lack self-control, but usually it's because they're too disciplined and constantly play the 'good girl' and need to create more space in their life for self-care," says Ali Shapiro, a top health coach based in Philadelphia. Self-care isn't always about bubble baths and massages. Sometimes it's about leaving the office at 5 p.m. or taking a lunch break.

"Eating fulfills the human need for comfort and pleasure," says Shapiro. If you're grinding out your days without room for even one activity that brings you pleasure, you might use food as a quick fix because it's a lot easier to have a few cookies at night than to figure out what's stressing you out at work or with your relationships, or how to reprioritize your time. By understanding what the problem is, you can make a real change.

Connecting to what feeds you emotionally is as important as what you eat, says Shapiro. It's harder to lose weight when you're stressed because you have fewer emotional reserves, are more likely to end up reaching for comfort food, and then are apt to beat yourself up for being "bad," so you start the cycle all over again. That's why it's important to include weight-loss rewards like sexy workout clothes (see page 93 for cute gear ideas) or a trip to the spa during the Cosmo Bikini Diet—rather than waiting until the end—because feeling good will help the weight melt away faster.

FIGURE OUT WHAT MOVES YOU

Spend some time seriously thinking about what makes you feel good. Deep down inside we all know what would work for us, but the stories we tell ourselves hold us back from achieving lasting weight loss. Maybe it's "I'll look like a slacker if I leave for an hour for lunch," and so you act like a martyr and eat at your desk day in and day out.

In order to have a slim body, you must feed your soul first. "Weight loss is an opportunity for a lighter life," says Shapiro. "Working through your emotional baggage gives you the confidence and feeling of control you were projecting onto weight loss and food, because you'll start living more in line with your priorities."

To pinpoint your emotional-eating triggers, keep an emotional food journal this week. In other words, when you're filling out your daily food journal to track what you eat, also start writing down your feelings surrounding eating. Start paying attention to how food makes you feel: Are you feeling bloated? Deprived? Do you have energy? Can you concentrate better? Once you learn to better tune in to your body, you'll have the tools you need to combat emotional eating in all different kinds of situations.

Journaling helps you notice when you're overeating and why. It might be that you reach for candy every time you fight with your mom to help you calm down. Or maybe you're running around all day long, and when you finally sit at night you fill the stillness by downing everything in your cupboard.

If that's the case, take time to reflect after dinner and answer these questions in your food journal: When I overate, how did I feel during, afterward, and now? Did anything specific happen to trigger me to soothe myself with food? You may be overeating to fill a void in yourself or because you're craving more pleasure.

FEED YOUR SOUL, NOT YOUR FACE

Becoming more aware of your triggers is a great first step to knowing how to address your emotions about food. Try these five exercises to conquer emotional eating once and for all.

1 **Practice eating mindfully.** You may be used to gulping down your lunch at your desk while firing off e-mails rather than really tasting your food. To remind yourself to eat with more attention, try this easy eating meditation:
◆ Focus on a small morsel, such as a raisin or nut, noticing its shape, size, color, texture, and scent.

◆ Place it on your tongue, enjoying the flavor and keeping it in your mouth for as long as you can, or for at least 20 seconds.

◆ Chew slowly; swallow.

By turning your focus inward and concentrating on sensations such as taste and smell, eating can feel like a whole new experience. You'll also enjoy your meal more and notice that you feel full faster than when chowing while multitasking. Practice eating slowly and really chewing every bite, and you'll be better in tune with your hunger and fullness cues over time. In fact, studies show that mindful eating can help you stop a binge, shed pounds, and reduce your BMI (or body mass index, a common tool for gauging obesity).

2 **Be prepared.** Once you've pinpointed your emotional-eating triggers and the times that you're most likely to overindulge, arm yourself with preportioned snacks that you package at the start of the day so you don't overdo it when those cravings inevitably strike. Try an apple with a single-serve packet of almond butter. Or, depending on your specific cravings, fill plastic baggies with 1 ounce whole grain crackers, 48 pistachios, or ¼ cup dried fruit, such as mango.

3 **Fit in more bliss.** "If you aren't living a joyful life—despite getting enough rest, watching what you eat, and exercising regularly—you won't be able to reach or sustain your happy weight," says Erin Cox, author of *One Hot Mama*. An easy way to add a little fun and joy to your life is by making sure you treat yourself to one (Un)Guilty Pleasure every single day.

DID YOU REALLY NEED THE STUFFED CRUST?

Online pizza orders have 6 percent more calories than in-person and phone orders do, according to a recent study. "Private settings lower our inhibitions," says lead researcher Ryan McDevitt, an assistant professor in the Simon School of Business at the University of Rochester. Make online ordering feel social by doing it in front of a friend—or even look at a picture of someone you know while you click.

4 **Pinpoint your passions.** If you realize you're overeating to fill empty space in your life, you may just be lacking in inspiration. Try giving yourself 15 minutes every night before you go to bed to flip through magazines and collect articles and pictures in an inspiration folder to help you figure out what really brings you satisfaction and joy. You might be reminded about how much you love fashion or taking pictures or discover that you want to try painting (plenty of studios offer painting classes with wine tastings, and it makes for a fun date). Find like-minded people in your area on MeetUp.com to help cultivate your passions.

5 **Show some body love.** "I believe that loving yourself and your body is such an important—and frequently overlooked—component of weight loss," says Cox. "When you convince yourself that you're heavy and loathsome by looking at your body with disgust and criticizing your belly rolls, then you will subconsciously self-sabotage to remain at a higher number on the scale."

Try reversing body-bashing thoughts by looking at yourself in the mirror and finding something you can appreciate about those parts you loathe. Like if you hate your thighs, remind yourself that they carried you across the finish line for a 5K race. "When you truly love yourself and accept your body, I promise that taking care of yourself and making the lifestyle changes necessary to reach your body's ideal weight will be infinitely easier," says Cox.

HOW TO DEAL WITH ANY EMOTION

Sure, journaling and becoming more aware of your feelings can put you on the path to conquering binges, as can learning to eat more mindfully. But what happens when you're in that moment where you'd rather lose yourself in a gooey, warm chocolate brownie with a glass of creamy milk than face the anger that comes with suspecting your BF is cheating on you or the stress from planning for a big work presentation? In those moments, taking a warm bath or calling a friend just isn't going to be able to stop you from resisting the instant gratification that comes from indulging in that pint of ice cream or bag of chips. Check out this real-world advice for better ways to deal with overpowering emotions.

Anger

"When you're angry, it's no surprise that you may want to reach for something crunchy like potato chips, nuts, and snack mix to satisfy that gnawing feeling," says Susan Albers, PsyD, a psychologist at the Cleveland Clinic and author of *Eating Mindfully*. "From a biological perspective, even animals bare their teeth and clench their jaws when angry or threatened."

Munching can be soothing and give you a release, so try a healthy alternative like baked tortilla chips with salsa, carrots dipped in hummus, or even licorice. Clenching and unclenching your jaw can help release some tension without consuming so many calories.

The alternative to eating: While you may be tempted to complain to a pal to let off steam, research shows that venting can sometimes make you dwell more rather than less. A better strategy is to find a release. "Distract yourself with another activity to get your mind off what's bothering you, such as taking a jog to burn off some adrenaline," says Dr. Albers.

Anxiety

Chocolate may be your go-to choice when you're feeling anxious. "Chocolate has many chemical properties that give us a little emotional buzz, such as a release of the feel-good chemicals dopamine and serotonin," says Dr. Albers. Instead of plowing through an entire plate of brownies, make chocolate pudding with fat-free milk or swap a milk chocolate candy bar for a glass of chocolate milk. See our other Bikini Diet sweet treats on page 182, like dark chocolate with strawberries or frozen mango with vanilla yogurt. Another soothing alternative could be chomping on icy foods, such as fruit Popsicles or frozen grapes.

The alternative to eating: "When you're anxious, your body moves into panic mode, where your heart beats faster and breathing quickens," says Dr. Albers. Studies show that yoga can help ease anxiety by bringing on a relaxation response through rhythmic movements and stretching, and the deep breathing used in the practice naturally helps slow an increased heart rate triggered by nervous energy. The next time you're anxious, try taking some deep breaths in child's pose where you sit on the floor with your knees bent and fold your chest and arms forward to channel stillness and peace.

Boredom

You may turn to foods you can munch mindlessly, such as popcorn or candy, when you're bored. Try eating something healthy with a spicy kick to keep your taste buds busy, like wasabi-flavored dry-roasted edamame or spicy hummus with veggies for dipping. "Not only does this give your mouth a kick, it can also wake up all of your senses so you're not zoning out," says Dr. Albers.

The alternative to eating: "Boredom eating is a big problem in our culture. With constant texting and browsing social media, it's hard to have a quiet moment without feeling the need to fill it in with an activity," says Dr. Albers. "Eating is entertaining and fills gaps in time." Instead of trying to find something to do during every single down moment, close your eyes, let your body completely relax, and simply stay still.

Happiness

Being happy can make you overeat too, since we use celebrations as a reason to indulge. Feeling good may trigger cravings for flavors linked with holidays and parties, such as apple pie and cake, because our brains associate them with happy times. If you're craving apple pie, bake a small apple and top it with 2 tablespoons low-fat plain yogurt sprinkled with cinnamon. You'll get the same tart taste sans the fatty butter from the crust.

The alternative to eating: "It's a myth that we only emotionally eat when we're sad, angry, or upset. Instead, we eat in response to *any* emotion, and sometimes we reach for food to try to hold on to feelings of joy for longer," says Dr. Albers. Try to find alternative ways to hold on to the pleasure, such as tweeting at friends to share the good times in your life.

Loneliness

Lonely people may tend to dive into a pint of ice cream to soothe themselves after, say, a breakup. "It may be because dairy has calming and sedative properties," says Dr. Albers. "It may also be a pop culture association that has evolved—almost every breakup movie features a woman eating ice cream right out of the carton."

The guilt that often follows a pint of ice cream doesn't do much to ease loneliness, so go for fat-free Greek yogurt instead. "It still provides comforting creaminess but also has protein, which is energizing, and less sugar, which keeps glucose levels steady," says Dr. Albers.

The alternative to eating: "We can't make food our primary relationship, so the only cure for loneliness is to find connection," says Dr. Albers. "If it's 2 a.m. and you can't call a friend, send someone you miss but who you've lost touch with a message on Facebook. You can also write a letter the old-fashioned way with paper and a pen, telling someone how much they mean to you." Focusing on gratitude and the people in your life whom you care about can help ease the urge to binge.

Sadness

Having the blues may make you more likely to reach for comfort foods that bring back happy memories from childhood, like mac and cheese. Instead, make whole wheat pasta with fat-free milk, low-fat extra-sharp cheese, and chopped broccoli. Using broccoli along with low-fat cheese cuts a whopping 300 calories and 26 grams of fat. Another traditional comfort food favorite is mashed potatoes, so make them healthier by boiling a small to medium potato until tender, draining, and mashing with 1 teaspoon of olive oil, a dash of garlic powder, and salt to taste. The dish is full of flavor without using butter!

The alternative to eating: Flipping through old photos to relive happy memories (think: your graduation party or spring break) may be a better pick-me-up than eating comfort food. When researchers looked at how much people's moods rose after eating a chocolate snack, sipping a cocktail, watching TV, listening to music, or looking at personal photos, they found the winner by a long shot was viewing pictures.

Stress

You probably tend to go for fatty and sugary foods when you're experiencing the S word because the release of cortisol sends your body into flight-or-fight mode, making you crave the energy that fatty foods like French fries and sugary foods provide.

"Foods that regulate your blood sugar are a must when you're stressed out," says Dr. Albers. "My favorite food for stress relief is pistachios because they help keep blood sugar levels steady for energy; are the type of nuts lowest in calories and fat; and buying them in shells makes you automatically slow down when you eat them so you don't consume as many."

The alternative to eating: Replace food with activities that naturally reduce your cortisol levels, such as taking a time-out to read with a soothing cup of black tea. A study in the journal *Psychopharmacology* found that drinking black tea reduces your cortisol levels by 47 percent. Bonus: Drinking tea or other healthy hydrators like water can also fill up your stomach so you ache less to fill it with food.

BIKINI DIET MEAL PLAN WEEK 4

Turn to the Month 1 Bikini Diet Meal Plan Cheat Sheet on page 22 for a quick overview on what to eat this week, or go to Chapter 14, page 163, for details on portion sizes and recipes. Remember, this week's eating goal is to focus on what's going on inside your head and your heart. Don't forget to write down how you feel about yourself and your meals in your food journal (or to take notes at the end of this chapter) to get a better idea of how your emotions might drive your appetite. Then write down concrete strategies on how you might feed your soul instead of your stomach for the next time you're faced with an emotional-eating trigger.

MOTIVATION IN YOUR MAILBOX

KlutchClub is a subscription-based service that delivers the latest fitness and health products to your door. Sign up (it's $16 a month) and get $50 worth of swag in the mail each month. Bonus: If you review the products on KlutchClub's website (KlutchClub.com), you receive points that can add up to a free box of goodies pretty quickly.

STAR-SPIRATION

Get fired up to slim down with these tips tweeted to **@Cosmopolitan** by Hollywood trainers. Even starlets need motivation!

"Commit 2 the process (not the scale). Break down steps u need 2 take each day. Did you walk 10,000 steps? Eat 5 times? Sleep 7-8 hrs?" **@HarleyPasternak** (Harley Pasternak, trainer to **Megan Fox** and **Sophia Bush**)

"Follow every lower-body exercise with a core move: sit-ups, crunches, twists, or a 45-sec plank. Every move, all year. Results motivate." **@Gunnar** (Gunnar Peterson, trainer to **Kim Kardashian** and **Sofia Vergara**)

"Pick activities you enjoy. If you love how you're spending your time, you'll have fun, keep going back for more, and get results!" **@TaraStiles** (Tara Stiles, trainer to **Brooklyn Decker** and **Tia Mowry**)

"Create a daily motivation mantra. something like 'My body is changing.' or 'Every obstacle is an opportunity.' **@MsMandyIngber** (Mandy Ingber, trainer to **Jennifer Aniston** and **Kate Beckinsale**)

HOT & HEALTHY WORKOUT WEEK 4

In the past 3 weeks, you've successfully kicked off a workout routine!

Here's what to do this week:

◆ Morning Cardio Blast, 4 to 5 times this week, as soon as you wake up (See page 201.)
◆ Tracy Anderson's Lean Thighs—No Lunges! toning routine, twice this week—but not on consecutive days! (See page 202.)
◆ Barry's Bootcamp Total-Body Strength Circuit, twice this week—but not on consecutive days! (See page 202.)
◆ Feel-Good Fitness day once this week (See page 203.)
◆ Rest and recover—2 days this week, but not on consecutive days!

Grab a chair for doing Tracy Anderson's Lean Thighs—No Lunges! routine and try these simple moves to tone and firm, just in time for shorts season. As you do each move, imagine someone is pulling your foot away from your body. That maximizes the stretch and actually lengthens your muscles.

"Now that you're really in the groove, focus on proper form during your strength-training sessions and visualize your end results," says Barry Jay of Barry's Bootcamp. Make sure you're measuring and recording your inches every week and that you've written down what you'd like your measurements to be at the end of the 12 weeks in your Happy Weight Goals section at the front of this book.

(UN)GUILTY PLEASURE: TAKE A LUNCH BREAK

This week, just say no to desktop dining. Most of us are guilty of chowing down inside our cubes: Eighty-three percent of Americans regularly eat at their desks, according to a survey by the American Dietetic Association and ConAgra Foods' Home Food Safety program.

Instead of eating your lunch in front of your computer, take a *real* lunch break. That means backing away from your desk and heading solo to a coffee shop; chilling out on a bench in a park with last night's leftovers; or joining coworkers at a laid-back restaurant. The key is to give yourself a mental break from work, to really focus on your food, and to fully chew each bite. This way you're nourishing your body and your emotions to ward off stress eating.

If you need even more motivation to break your desktop-dining habit, chew on this: A study by the University of Arizona found the average desktop has 100 times more bacteria than a kitchen table and 400 times more than the average toilet seat. It may sound bogus, but one possible reason may be because you clean your toilet and kitchen more than you clean your workspace.

Try eating lunch away from your desk every day this week (even if you can escape for only 25 or 30 minutes), and pay attention to how taking a lunch break made you feel. Do you have more energy? Can you concentrate better?

Not only will you feel more productive when you get back in the office, but you'll also probably eat less later on. That's because it's hard to enjoy your food when you're scarfing it down in your fluorescent-lit cubicle while pounding out an email. And if you're not getting emotional pleasure from food, then you won't feel satiated and you'll be more likely to reach for a candy bar at 3 p.m.

SUCCESS TRACKER:

Bikini Body Checklist Week 4

☐ I've kept an emotional food journal to help me better recognize my emotional-eating triggers, and have tried other ways to soothe myself besides turning to food for a quick fix.

☐ I've tried eating more mindfully with an eating meditation at least once a day this week.

☐ I've followed the Bikini Diet meal plan.

☐ I've followed the Hot & Healthy Workout plan.

☐ I've eaten lunch away from my desk every single day this week—even if I could get away for only 20 minutes. I noted how it made me feel in my food diary or the space below.

Week 4 Measurements

Weight _____

Waist _____

Chest _____

Hips _____

This week I feel _____

_____

_____

_____

_____

_____

_____

_____

_____

_____

_____

_____

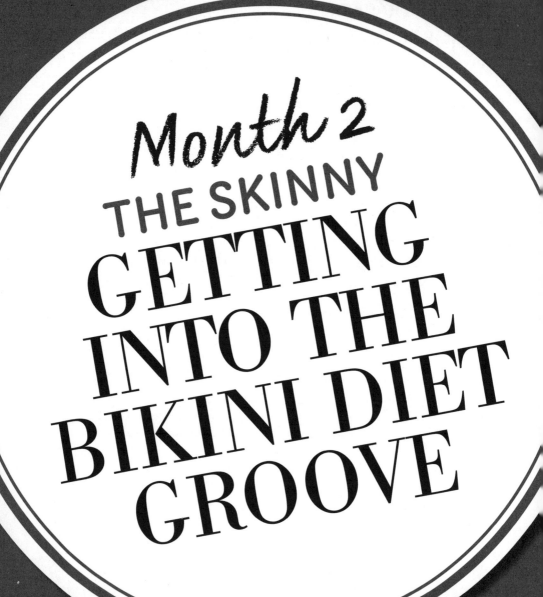

Month 2

THE SKINNY

GETTING INTO THE BIKINI DIET GROOVE

YOU GO, GIRL! You have successfully completed 4 weeks of the Cosmo Bikini Diet. Your clothes are a little looser, and you may be feeling lighter and more energetic. During the next month, consistency is the name of the game. A new meal plan will keep you from getting stuck in a food rut, and Barry's Bootcamp is switching things up with a different strength-training workout (hint: you'll need those resistance bands now).

If you're feeling discouraged because the weight doesn't seem to be coming off as fast as you'd like, then the cause might be stress. After all, stress *can* make you fat. That's why if you're not fitting enough pleasure into your day—despite eating healthy and working out regularly—you won't be able to score your sexiest bikini body. It sounds strange, but happiness may actually be a weight-loss wonder: Worms given a boost of serotonin, a chemical linked to improved mood, slashed their fat levels by up to 50 percent, finds a study in *Cell Metabolism*. Researchers speculate that serotonin signals the brain to speed up metabolism, which blocks fat storage in both worms and humans alike.

So if happiness makes you skinnier, how does chronic stress make you pack on the pounds? When you're anxious, your body registers it as famine and is less efficient at processing sugar and fat, so your metabolism may slow down and fat clings to you, making it tougher to shed pounds. That's why stress throws a wrench in the whole "calories in and calories out" concept.

And while you can try to combat angst in the moment, it's not like you can totally eliminate the S word from your life. Some stress is actually good for you because it gives you energy and forces you to take action—such as having an all-night brainstorming session for a big presentation. But if you're eating unsatisfying diet food, killing yourself at the gym for hours a day, and logging 12 more at the office, that surge in cortisol triggered by your demanding life is going to make getting that bikini body all the more challenging. **We are here to remind you that weight loss doesn't have to be torturous or feel like a deprivation diet**—and that by allowing yourself little pleasures every single day, you'll actually score a healthier, sexier body than by kicking your own butt trying to slim down.

While you can't realistically tell your boss you're going to start working from home or make that hot guy you're dating less of a commitment-phobe, you *can* create room for moments of fun every single day. What feels like a treat or brings joy is different for every woman, but for you it might mean calling your funniest friend for a few minutes at the end of a killer day at the office; putting your feet up to read gossip mags with a glass of wine; or skipping laundry chores to hit your favorite yoga class. That's why incorporating the (Un)Guilty Pleasure suggestions each week is just as important to achieving your sexy bikini body as are eating healthy and working out.

Read on for the details to uncover even more secrets to bring you closer to your happy weight and your sexiest body ever.

BIKINI DIET MEAL PLA

day	BREAKFAST	SNACK	LUNCH
1	Waffle & eggs (p. 170); fruit; coffee or tea	Turkey & cheese roll-ups (p. 175); fruit; coffee or tea	Almond butter and pear sandwich (p. 171); dry-roasted edamame; red bell pepper slices w hummus; seltzer water
2	Cottage cheese & berries (p. 170); coffee or tea	Hard-boiled egg; apple (p. 175)	Turkey sub or sandwich (p. 171); carrots & hummus (p. 171); grapes; seltzer water
3	Blueberry chia smoothie (p. 170); coffee or tea	Raisins & peanuts or other nut (like almonds or cashews) (p. 175)	Black bean soup w/crackers (p. 171); cheese; fruit
4	Mango-coconut oatmeal (p. 170); coffee or tea	Apple slices w/ almond butter or other nut butter (p. 176)	Hummus & cucumber pita sandwich (p. 171); sliced strawberries; seltzer water
5	Avocado smoothie (p. 170); almonds; coffee or tea	Whole wheat crackers w/cheese (p. 176)	Thai chopped chicken salad (p. 172); apple; unsweetened tea
6	Scrambled eggs & spinach (p. 171); whole wheat toast; coffee or tea	Sliced red bell peppers; whole wheat pretzels; Greek yogurt dip (p. 176)	Cranberry crunch yogurt parfait (p. 172); seltzer water
7	EARNED DAY ⟶ (page 34)		

WEEKLY AVERAGE DAILY NUTRITION FACTS:
About 1,500 calories plus 150 Flex Calories for about 1,650 calories total, 50 g total fat, 13 g saturated fat, 0 g trans fat, 11 g monounsatur ed fat, 5 g polyunsaturated fat, 219 mg choles terol, 2,549 mg sodium, 193 g carbs, 30 g fibe

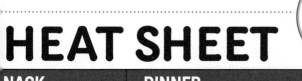

HEAT SHEET

WEEKS
5-8

NACK	DINNER	FLEX CALORIES
ips w/ salsa (p. 175)	Macadamia-crusted tilapia w/pineapple salsa (p. 172); sesame snow peas (p. 173); milk or milk substitute	150 calories to spend as you like
nana slices w/pea- butter (p. 175)	Wonton soup and teriyaki soba noodle bowl (p. 173)	150 calories to spend as you like
na & celery 175)	Grilled pork tenderloin w/ roasted grapes (p. 173); sesame snow peas (p. 173); brown rice	Strawberry waffle sundae dessert (p. 175) or 150 calories to spend as you like
ia seed pudding 176)	Tropical mahi mahi salad (p. 174); baked sweet potato (p. 179); milk or milk substitute	150 calories to spend as you like
real & fruit 176)	Pot stickers w/ ginger-lemon dipping sauce (p. 174); Asian vegetables (p. 174); edamame (p. 174); milk or milk substitute	150 calories to spend as you like
eese & pear 176)	Flatbread asparagus pizza (p. 175); strawberry spinach salad (p. 175); milk or milk substitute	Light ice cream with fruit (p. 176) or 150 calories to spend as you like

0 g sugar, 85 g protein. Ratio of calories from
arbohydrates, protein, and fat: 50% carbohy-
rates, 20% protein, and 30% fat.

HOT & HEALTHY FITNESS PROGRAM WEEKS 5-8

At this point you're already feeling stronger and fitter, as well as more energetic. In the coming weeks, you'll build on the program you've successfully mastered in the first month. There's a fun new 15-minute Morning Cardio Blast routine to try each week. Also to keep shaking things up, you'll be doing a new Barry's Bootcamp Rubber Band Workout twice a week (see page 205). Do this eight-move exercise circuit twice in a row (and take 30 seconds of recovery in between each move) for an all-over toning workout in only about 25 minutes! Doing different strength moves than in the first month challenges your body to give you extra definition that you'll love showing off on the beach.

And you'll still get the 6-minute targeted toning sessions from Tracy Anderson, also twice a week. You'll continue to enjoy one Feel-Good Fitness day plus two days off every week so your muscles can recover.

Month 2

HOT & HEALTHY
WORKOUT CHEAT SHEET

You'll find instructions for all the routines in Chapter 15.

DAY	WORKOUT	MINUTES
1	Morning Cardio Blast (pages 205, 209, 212, 215) Tracy Anderson's Toning Routine (pages 207, 210, 213, 216)	15 6
	TOTAL WORKOUT TIME	**21**
2	Morning Cardio Blast (pages 205, 209, 212, 215) Barry's Bootcamp Rubber Band Workout (pages 205, 209, 212, 215)	15 25
	TOTAL WORKOUT TIME	**40**
3	Rest and recover!	
4	Morning Cardio Blast (pages 205, 209, 212, 215) Tracy Anderson's Toning Routine (pages 207, 210, 213, 216)	15 6
	TOTAL WORKOUT TIME	**21**
5	Morning Cardio Blast (pages 205, 209, 212, 215) Barry's Bootcamp Rubber Band Workout (pages 205, 209, 212, 215)	15 25
	TOTAL WORKOUT TIME	**40**
6	Rest and recover!	
7	Morning Cardio Blast (Optional) (pages 205, 209, 212, 215) Feel-Good Fitness day (pages 209, 211, 214, 217)	15 30-45
	TOTAL WORKOUT TIME	**45-60**

CHAPTER FIVE

SNACK TO LOSE

WEEK #5

THE LOWDOWN So far the Cosmo Bikini Diet should not feel like a diet, because each of our meal plans includes plenty of snacks to keep you full. This week is no exception!

We show you how to eat *more* in order to lose; why eating every 4 hours can actually cut overall calorie consumption; and we'll give you healthy-but-yummy food swaps to satisfy your cravings even when those cookies are just screaming your name.

Now that you're into the second month of the plan, we'll also share a secret about how to overcome a weight-loss plateau for when the scale gets stuck. Plus, find out which processed foods you should ditch right now to avoid bikini-bod sabotage and how a daily chocolate fix can help you slim down (really!). Melting away your belly fat never tasted so good!

THE RULES OF SMART SNACKING

You might think that skipping snacks is a surefire way to slash extra calories so you slim down faster. While it makes sense in theory, research shows that people who report eating at least four times a day (as opposed to eating three or less) are actually slimmer. Why? It could be because waiting too long to eat between meals as opposed to deliberately sitting down for a legit snack means you're instead taking little nibbles here and there that you're not counting as calories but that add up big-time. A sneaky muffin-top culprit might be those mindless bites.

Or it might be that forgoing snacks between meals means you've gone for such a long stretch without eating anything at all that when mealtime finally *does* roll around, your out-of-control hunger pangs prompt you to scarf down so much food that you feel like you have to roll yourself away from the table.

Let's say it's been 4 hours since you had breakfast, so you absent-mindedly dip into the candy bowl at work as you walk by and grab two handfuls of M&Ms. That's an extra 60 calories a day. It doesn't sound like much, but it adds up to 21,900 calories over the course of a year—or an extra 6 pounds (that's enough to build a spare tire around your waist).

Or say you had a virtuous salad for dinner while your BF had pizza, and you've sworn off postmeal snacks. Still, you munch on the two crusts left over on his plate as you're cleaning up—that's an extra 130 calories! You could have treated yourself to 2 cups of fresh strawberries with a square of dark chocolate for about the same calorie count... and felt more satisfied.

On the other hand, maybe you have iron willpower and can avoid munching on even a teeny-tiny bite between meals all day. Then the waitress brings over a warm, crusty bread bowl at 7 p.m. and your rumbling stomach prompts you to dive in for a feel-good carb fix. Just a few soft, doughy slices dipped in olive oil and sprinkled with sea salt may cost you about 350 calories—and that's *before* you've even ordered an appetizer, entrée, or glass of wine.

We know, all this calorie talk is probably making your head spin. We're not telling you to vigilantly count calories (that goes against the Cosmo Bikini Diet Pledge!). Instead what we're saying is that by learning to pay more attention to all those little bites and listen to your hunger cues by allowing yourself small, satiating snacks, you'll shed weight without feeling deprived.

THE 4 RULES THAT WILL HELP YOU LOSE MORE BY SNACKING OFTEN

1 **Go for whole foods.** Snacking can help you slim down by keeping blood sugar levels steady so you don't unconsciously munch or overindulge at lunch and dinner—as long as you eat real, whole food. While low-calorie energy bars, chips, and other processed foods may be convenient, most are also low in skin-beautifying antioxidants and filling fiber and may be high in sodium (which causes belly bloat!). Plan ahead by having snack options on hand that are heavy on fruits or veggies and light on processed ingredients. Produce-rich snacks that don't take time to prepare include:

◆ ½ cup salsa with 1 ounce whole grain crackers (see page 88.)
◆ ½ cup cherry tomatoes or baby carrots with 2 teaspoons hummus (see page 180.)
◆ ¼ cup dried apricots and 1 tablespoon sunflower seeds (see page 169.)
◆ Pear with a part-skim mozzarella cheese stick (see page 182.)
◆ ½ cup low-fat cottage cheese with 1 sliced kiwifruit (see page 169.)
◆ Also see the pre- and postworkout snack ideas on page 49-50.

2 **Balance your snacks.** To keep your blood sugar steady, make sure that every snack includes the healthy trifecta of protein, whole grains, and healthy fats (each of the above examples has all three). Fiber-rich or nutrient-dense snacks (fruits, nuts, low-fat cheese) are longer-lasting pick-me-ups than the sugar- and fat-filled treats we tend to yearn for (chips! cookies! ice cream!), so you're apt to eat less overall—and have stronger willpower when your coworker walks by with a plate of her addictive brownies.

3 **Practice portion control.** While you may already know that eating often can help you lose more weight by revving your metabolism, remember the Cosmo Bikini Diet Secret in Week 1 that overdoing it on even healthy foods can make for unnecessary calories—and added belly fat. Portion-size snacks help you tame your appetite without going overboard with fat and calories. Like if you decide to have almonds as a snack, stick to a shot glass' worth (or 22 almonds) rather than robotically feeding your face with five or six big handfuls. Or preportion trail mix by dividing ¼-cup servings into small plastic baggies ahead of time. Toss one into your purse before you walk out the door so you have a healthy, portion-controlled option on hand when hunger strikes.

4 **Timing matters.** Eat roughly every 4 hours to keep energy levels stable and to help ward off junk food cravings. Having an afternoon snack suggested in each monthly meal plan should be like meeting your friends for weekly happy hour—something you won't miss—since the stretch between lunch and dinner can feel like forever.

RECORD EVERY BITE TO HURDLE A WEIGHT-LOSS PLATEAU

If you've banned afternoon trips to the vending machine, followed the Hot & Healthy Workout plans, and *still* aren't seeing the pounds melt away, the culprit could be small stuff that you're not even thinking about. That's why keeping your food diary is so important. If you're finding that you've hit a weight-loss plateau and can't figure out why, make sure you're being *totally* honest with yourself and recording every little extra lick of peanut butter or bite of pizza crust. You may be surprised to find that when you truly record every nibble, your mindless

MAKE SMART SWAPS TO SATISFY CRAVINGS

Whether you crave sweet, salty, crunchy, or savory snacks, or even a combination, there are times when your body simply needs an energy boost. Try these healthy snack options:

Creamy
◆ Laughing Cow Light cheese wedge spread with sliced cucumbers
◆ ½ cup low-fat yogurt with 2 tablespoons sugar-free jam

Crunchy
◆ Dip carrots, sliced bell peppers, and sugar snap peas in 2 tablespoons hummus or guacamole
◆ 1 ounce black bean tortilla chips with ½ cup salsa

Salty
◆ ½ cup shelled edamame with sea salt
◆ 1 cup miso soup
◆ 22 roasted and salted almonds

Savory
◆ Combine 2 ounces water-packed tuna with 2 tablespoons Dijon mustard
◆ Mix together 2 hard-boiled diced egg whites, diced celery, and 2 tablespoons light mayo

Sweet
◆Warm up half a ripe banana, 1 square chocolate, ¼ cup oats, and a drizzle honey; top with sliced almonds and mash together

munching could add up to a whole other meal. Let's do the math:
◆ 2 handfuls of M&Ms = 60 calories
◆ 2 pizza crusts that your BF left in the box = 130 calories
◆ 10 french fries from your friend's plate at lunch (hey, you didn't order them, so you didn't think they counted enough to write in your food diary) = 93 calories
◆ A few extra licks of peanut or almond butter left over on the knife after you made your sandwich for lunch as suggested on day 1 of this month's meal plan = 165 calories
◆ Total mindless calories munched = 448 calories, or enough food to equal an extra meal!

◆ Blend together ½ frozen banana with ½ cup low-fat coconut milk for a smoothie
◆ Make a parfait by layering ½ cup diced pineapple with ½ cup low-fat Greek yogurt in a clear glass

Sweet and Salty
◆ Make trail mix popcorn by mixing together 1 cup air-popped popcorn, 1 teaspoon dried cranberries, and 1 teaspoon chocolate chips
◆ 24 shelled pistachios with a small box of raisins

PROCESSED FOODS TO DITCH RIGHT NOW

These packaged eats may be bad for your waistline and your health. Here are the ones to skip and easy ideas for nutritious swaps.

Packaged Egg Whites

It's better to eat the real deal, because those egg-white substitutes often contain artificial ingredients such as "color" and "maltodextrin" (a sweetener also used in candy). Plus you might want to ditch egg-white omelets. Remember: Egg yolks are important sources of nutrients that boost memory, keep fat from building up in your liver, and make up your cell membranes (see page 42).

Healthier swap: Make a batch of protein-rich hard-boiled eggs ahead of time so you can just grab and go in the morning with a piece of fruit. Place a few eggs in a saucepan, fill it with cold water so the tops of the eggs are covered by about an inch of liquid, and bring it to a boil. As soon as it starts to boil, reduce the heat and let it simmer for about a minute. Take the pan off the stove, cover, and let sit for about 10 to 12 minutes. Place the eggs in ice water until cool. You can then store them in the refrigerator in a covered container for up to 5 days.

Flavored Chips

People who regularly eat foods with the flavor enhancer monosodium glutamate, or MSG, are three times more likely to be overweight than those who don't—even if their calorie intake and physical activity are equal, finds a study in the journal *Obesity*. MSG isn't found only in Chinese food, but also in many snack foods like flavored chips.

Healthier swap: The best way to avoid MSG is to eat as many whole, unprocessed foods as you can, since MSG isn't usually listed on food labels—and even packaged foods that say *no MSG added* may still have the flavor enhancer. For example, if you're craving something cheese flavored, use shredded Cheddar, or try sprinkling spices in hummus or Greek yogurt to make a flavorful, healthy dip for veggies.

Fat-Free Potato Chips

Many fat-free chips are made with Olestra, an ingredient whose side effects include diarrhea (definitely not something you want to deal with during bikini season). Plus, chips are low in fiber, so one measly serving won't fill you up, and you'll be likely to reach for more or overeat later.

Healthier swap: For a crunchy snack, go for popcorn instead. You can have 3 cups of air-popped popcorn for only about 100 calories (try spicing it up by sprinkling with garlic salt). It's also packed with filling fiber and disease-fighting antioxidants.

Instant Oatmeal

Those little packets of instant oatmeal cook so quickly because they're processed, which means they have a high glycemic index, so your body also digests them quickly. Translation: You'll be reaching for a midmorning snack to tide you over well before lunch.
Healthier swap: Slow-cooked oats take longer to make, but they are also less processed, have a low glycemic index, and will leave you feeling full until lunch. To save time, make a batch of steel-cut oats on the weekends and then divide it into portion-controlled containers to use in delicious breakfasts through the week (see page 42).

Canned Soups, Fruits, and Veggies

Canned foods may be convenient, but eating too many of them is a prime culprit for water retention and tummy bloat because they're often loaded with extra sodium.
Healthier swap: To reduce your added sodium intake, limit the amount of canned foods you eat by instead choosing vegetables and soups in plastic bags or pouches like Tabatchnick vegetable soup; try to eat fresh whenever possible.

Salad Dressings

You might want to skip the processed dressings when it comes to flavoring your salad, because they're often packed with added sugars, and the light varieties tend to have the most in an attempt to cover up the low-fat taste.
Healthier swap: Try mixing up your own by following the Healthy Balsamic Dressing recipe from Jonathan Rollo of Greenleaf Chopshop in Los Angeles on page 165. You can make it ahead of time and just store it in the fridge to spice up salads and veggies.

Diet Soda

While some caffeine is good for you (see page 43), there's about as much caffeine in one can of Diet Coke as there is in a shot of espresso, so having a few cans a day could leave you feeling high and then low when you come down from the caffeine buzz. Besides triggering major dips in energy, reaching for cans as a pick-me-up makes it tougher to fall asleep in the normal 30-minute range come bedtime. (See page 36 on the slimming benefits of a good night's sleep.) Plus, the acidity in soda can damage tooth enamel if sipped daily.
Healthier swap: Go for natural berry-flavored seltzer water for a fizz sans caffeine and chemicals. Or try adding sliced cucumbers to give plain old water a kick. Bonus: It will

keep you hydrated to help ward off thirst-induced hunger binges later on. See page 19 for more ways to make plain old water more flavorful.

Sugar-Free Bars

Sorbitol, an artificial sweetener found in many sugar-free products, is difficult for your body to break down and can cause bloating and indigestion.

Healthier swap: For a more nutritious go-to snack, keep naturally-low-in-sugar bars on hand that have fewer than five ingredients. A delicious option: the Dark Chocolate Nuts & Sea Salt from KIND Bar. It tastes indulgent but has only 5 grams of sugar. Plus, the bar is high in both satiating fiber (7 grams) and protein (6 grams). It tastes so good, you won't be tempted to raid the vending machine for a candy bar fix.

Low-Fat Frozen Dinners

Relying on these seemingly diet-friendly meals in place of fresh, whole foods could actually sabotage your stay-slim efforts. Eating a lot of fat-free and low-fat foods is apt to leave you unsatisfied and craving something more substantial, so you reach for a late-night snack.

Healthier swap: Try mixing tuna fish with greens and 2 tablespoons olive oil and balsamic vinegar dressing, and adding a side of steamed mixed veggies (we like the Birds Eye Steamfresh bags) tossed with sliced almonds for a more nutritious dinner packed with healthy fats.

BIKINI DIET MEAL PLAN WEEK 5

Turn to the Month 2 Bikini Diet Meal Plan Cheat Sheet on page 72 for a quick overview on what to eat this week, or go to Chapter 14, page 170, for details on portion sizes and recipes. One of the best parts of the Cosmo Bikini Diet is that you don't have to starve to slim down. Snacking makes you skinnier by controlling appetite, so don't try to fast between meals. If your stomach is rumbling, grab any of the portion-controlled snack ideas such as an apple with almond butter or raisins and peanuts, outlined in the monthly meal plans, to tide you over until your next meal.

HOT & HEALTHY WORKOUT WEEK 5

Congratulations! You've completed a whole month of Bikini Diet workouts.

Here's what to do this week:

◆ Morning Cardio Blast, 4 to 5 times this week, as soon as you wake up (See page 205.)
◆ Barry's Bootcamp Rubber Band Workout, twice this week—but not on consecutive days! (See page 205.)
◆ Tracy Anderson's Cellulite-Zapping Workout, twice this week—but not on consecutive days! (See page 207.)

- Feel-Good Fitness day once this week (See page 209.)
- Rest and recover—2 days this week, but not on consecutive days!

This week you can start to zap those pesky lumps with four cellulite-zapping moves from Tracy Anderson in only 6 minutes. They're designed to tighten your muscle fibers, so you'll look toned and smooth. Each time you do this routine, complete it in a different order to keep your muscles guessing. It makes the exercises even more effective.

"Now your goal is to maintain consistency by keeping it going and sticking to a new set schedule," says Barry Jay of Barry's Bootcamp. "This month, we leave the weights behind and take it up a notch by introducing resistance bands, or in layman's terms, a rubber band workout! These bands come in varying levels of resistance, and choosing the right one is very important." Start with your lighter resistance band for phase 1, or the first 2 weeks of month 2. (See page 11 for guidelines on getting the right resistance band.) Be sure that your resistance bands feel challenging, because that will make your body work harder for faster sculpting results. You'll be toning up all over in just about 25 minutes with this fun routine.

(UN)GUILTY PLEASURE: SLIM DOWN WITH CHOCOLATE

It may sound too good to be true, but a study shows that regular chocolate eaters are actually slimmer than people who don't indulge as often—even though they ate slightly more calories overall and did not exercise any longer than the control group. Savoring the sweet stuff may be not only a metabolism booster, but also a mood booster: Eating chocolate can make you happy because it increases levels of the feel-good hormones known as serotonin and dopamine in your brain.

That doesn't mean that ripping open the wrapper on a supersized candy bar is going to burn belly fat (all those sugar-filled empty calories will only expand your waistline) or give you a happiness high (more likely it'll make you feel guilty for overindulging). However, treating yourself to a square or two of *dark* chocolate most days will be better for your bikini body than swearing it off completely, because you'll get a feel-good buzz and help tame a sweet tooth. The secret is to go for the real, unprocessed kind that's at least 70 percent dark chocolate. (If you see cacao on the ingredient list, it's just referring to the bean that chocolate and cocoa are made from.) One reason dark is better than milk or white is because it has a lot less added sugar, which means it won't send your blood sugar (and energy levels) suddenly rising and then crashing—which gives you the opposite of a mood boost. It's also higher in age-fighting antioxidants known as flavonoids.

This week, try spending your daily Flex Calories on a few squares of the sweet dark stuff. To make your daily chocolate fix feel completely pampering, eat it when you can sit down and focus fully on relaxing and tasting this sweet treat. If you saved it for after dinner, put on your coziest pair of PJs, chill out to a calming soundtrack, maybe light some candles. Hey, it works to get you in the mood for sex, so why not make indulging your sweet tooth just as sensual? Then slowly unwrap your chocolate and savor each delicious bite. This small move will definitely *not* make you forget you're on a "diet." Who knew getting in bikini shape could taste so good?

Here are some delicious, healthy picks to look for:

Trader Joe's 72% Cacao Dark Chocolate You can eat half of this creamy, coffeelike bar for 140 rich calories, and you'll also get 3 grams of fiber.

Organic Dark Chocolate Covered Cacao Nibs These little flavor bursts from Kopali Organics are made from bits of the beans where chocolate comes from to satisfy both sweet and crunchy cravings. They're vegan and fair trade, and have only 140 calories per serving.

Next Organics Dark Chocolate Almonds Coated with 70 percent cacao dark chocolate, these crunchy almonds are packed with healthy fats and vitamin E for lustrous skin and hair.

Vega Maca Chocolate Bar Maca powder is made from a plant root touted for its energy- and libido-enhancing powers. This gluten-free bar is made with 70 percent dark chocolate cacao.

Endangered Species Dark Chocolate Squares If you can't trust yourself to eat just one or two pieces, go for these decadent, individually wrapped dark chocolate squares for about only 50 calories each and automatic portion control. Pop two for a 100-calorie treat.

SUCCESS TRACKER:

Bikini Body Checklist Week 5

☐ I've snacked smart by:

    ☐ Munching on whole foods that combine protein, whole grain carbs, and healthy fats

    ☐ Paying attention to portion sizes

    ☐ Making sure to eat about every 4 hours

☐ I've written down *everything* in my food dairy—even the tiny bites.

☐ I've made smart food swaps to help satisfy my cravings.

☐ I've replaced unhealthy processed foods with convenient, whole-food snacks.

☐ I've followed the Bikini Diet meal plan.

☐ I've followed the Hot & Healthy Workout plan.

Week 5 Measurements

Weight _____

Waist _____

Chest _____

Hips _____

This week I feel _____

_____

_____

_____

_____

_____

_____

_____

_____

_____

_____

CHAPTER SIX

FILL UP ON THE RIGHT CARBS

WEEK #6

THE LOWDOWN Congratulations! You're nearly halfway done with the 12-week program! Your tummy is tighter, and your energy levels are up. You're getting closer than ever to your sexiest bikini body, so keep up the good work.

If you want to lose weight without suffering from hunger pains, have at least 30 grams of fiber a day from high-quality carbs, such as whole grains, beans, fruits, and veggies. (If you're following the Bikini Diet meal plans, we have you covered—but a typical American woman gets only 13 grams a day!) We know, you've heard all about fiber, and it probably makes you think about prunes, regularity, and your grandma, but the truth is that making this one simple diet tweak can help you drop pounds without feeling like you want to chew your arm off. Here's why:

1. Fiber-rich foods have bulk so they fill you up faster and make you less likely to overeat.

2. Fiber-rich foods also tend to be low-calorie options. That means that you don't have to eat less to lose weight, but may actually be able to eat *more*!

3. Fiber triggers the release of the "I'm satisfied" hunger hormone and keeps blood sugar levels steady to help ward off cravings for unhealthy, fatty foods.

4. Adding more fiber to your diet also increases the amount of healthy bacteria in your gut, according to research from the University of Illinois. Having a healthy mix of gut bacteria not only boosts your immune system, but it also wards off weight gain to help you get your best bikini bod (more on this in Chapter 10 on page 132).

This week, you'll learn how to easily fill up on fiber by decoding labels and following the weekly meal plan. Don't skip the (Un)Guilty Pleasure—not only is it your reward for making it to the halfway milestone, but it will also keep you motivated to keep up with your workouts. You'll be confidently strutting your bikini body on the beach in no time.

KEEP YOUR FIBER FRESH

The Atkins days of living on meat and cheese are so over. You don't have to swear off carbs to shed inches around your middle—you just have to eat the right type. That means the kind that's loaded with fiber.

Dieters who cut 500 calories and got their carbs from only fiber-filled whole grains (think: rice) lost about twice as much belly fat as those who cut the same number of calories but ate only refined carbs (think: white bread), finds the *American Journal of Clinical Nutrition*. Experts think that eating fiber-heavy whole grains reduces glucose and insulin levels, which somehow alters fat metabolism to ward off jiggle around your middle.

So what are refined carbs, exactly? They're foods that aren't in their whole, natural form and that have additives, preservatives, and added fillers. Plus, refined carbs typically are made with white flour that has been stripped of fiber and other key nutrients. You'll usually find them in a box, bag, or wrapper. (Hint: If you can't pronounce an ingredient on the label, it's probably not natural and you might want to leave it on the grocery-store shelf.)

While many packaged foods boast high fiber on their labels, it's usually better to stick to the natural form over a processed one (think: rice versus rice cakes). And just because an ice cream bar has added fiber doesn't turn it into a health food, since not all fiber is created equal. Getting added fiber from packaged foods like yogurt and cookies probably won't offer the same health-boosting benefits as eating the unprocessed, intact kind found in whole grains, beans, and produce, according to the Center for Science in the Public Interest. If you can't give up packaged cookies, go for ones that list whole grains on the ingredient list to satisfy your sweet tooth *and* get a fiber fix. One to try: Kashi Oatmeal Raisin Flax cookies, which boast 4 grams of fiber from natural ingredients such as raisins, sunflower seeds, cranberries, shredded coconut, peanuts, almonds, walnuts, and flaxseeds.

Though all fiber counts look the same on nutrition labels, most processed fibers—such as inulin and maltodextrin—are finely ground, so they don't have the gummy texture or bulk that helps intact fiber slow digestion, lower cholesterol, and make you regular. Another type of added fiber, polydextrose, which is often found in foods like fat-free chips, may help keep you regular, but if you have a sensitive stomach, you'll also likely get gas and bloating. Your best bet is to stick to natural sources (think: fruits, veggies, and whole grains) to score your 30 grams a day.

Filling up on natural sources such as veggies means you'll automatically eat less. Why? First: Veggies are low-calorie fiber powerhouses. Second: They're also high in magnesium, which plays a big part in carbohydrate metabolism to help regulate blood sugar, which also keeps you from overeating. Here are three easy ways to get your fix.

1. Have a cup of vegetable soup before lunch. Both the fiber and water-based broth fill you up, leaving less space for snacks.

2. Add a side dish of Brussels sprouts to your dinner. Not only are they high in filling fiber (a cup has 4 grams and just 56 calories) but they're also packed with high levels of vitamins A and C, rank as a decent source of calcium, and are a proven skin rejuvenator. You may have gagged at these as a kid, but it's time to give them another try. This crunchy veg complements any meal. Sauté them with olive oil, pecans, and salt and pepper and they'll taste great.

3. Snack on salsa. Up your veggie and fiber intake by munching on ½ cup salsa with 1 ounce whole grain crackers.

Just a word of warning: If you've been on the low end of the fiber scale and up your intake too fast, it could cause gas and bloating (definitely not great for bikini season). So start slowly by incorporating more fruits and veggies and cutting back on packaged carbs. To help cut down on the bloating, drink plenty of water and try chewing some fennel seeds for gas relief.

GIVE YOUR CARBS A HIGH-FIBER MAKEOVER

Here's the Cosmo *Cliff's Notes* version for decoding nutrition labels and getting closer to your goal of 30 grams a day.

Instead of . . . white bread, tortilla, or pita
Try . . . whole grain bread, tortilla, or pita that has no more than 120 calories per serving and at least 3 grams of fiber. Just beware of sneaky labels and skip breads touting themselves as "whole grain" but that list highly processed, unbleached enriched wheat flour as one of the first ingredients. Instead, look for whole wheat flour as the first ingredient. Or better yet, choose breads that list plain ol' whole wheat, whole barley, whole millet, whole spelt, and other unprocessed, whole grain ingredients. Can you see little bits and pieces of grain in the slices? That's your clue that your slice hasn't been stripped of the good stuff.

Decode the label...Check out the label for Ezekiel 4:9 Sprouted Whole Grain Bread and you'll see that each slice has 80 calories and 3 grams of fiber per slice and is made with organic sprouted wheat, barley, millet, lentils, soybeans, and spelt. On the other hand, Wonder White Bread with Fibre has 95 calories and only 1.5 grams of fiber per slice, and the first three ingredients are unbleached wheat flour (NOT a whole grain!), water, and sugar. This bread is a health food imposter, while the ingredient list for the Ezekiel kind shows you that you're getting the most whole, filling fiber.

Instead of...cereal packed with empty calories, added sugar, or processed fiber
Try...cereal made with real, whole grains that have fewer than 180 calories per cup (be sure to read the label, because many cereals call a measly ½ cup one portion), less than 10 grams of sugar, and at least 5 grams of fiber.
Decode the label...If you compare the labels of Kashi's GoLean and Frosted Flakes, you'll see that Kashi Go Lean has 140 calories, 6 grams of sugar, and 10 grams of fiber in 1 cup. On the other hand, Kellogg's Frosted Flakes has 110 calories, 11 grams of sugar, and less than 1 gram of fiber per ¾ cup. Plus, Kashi's GoLean lists healthy whole grains like soy grits, hard red wheat, brown rice, whole grain oats, and barley at the top of its ingredients. Corn flakes? The main ingredients are milled corn and sugar—which are sure to send you reaching for a candy bar for an energy boost well before lunch.
Tip: If your whole grain breakfast cereal has at least 5 grams of fiber and you top it with a cup of blackberries or raspberries for an extra 8 grams, you've already met nearly half of your daily fiber goals at breakfast.

Q. HOW CAN I AVOID FEELING SLUGGISH AFTER A MEAL?

A. That woozy, drowsy feeling usually means you've eaten too much. When you overindulge, blood flow to your stomach increases, leaving less blood making its way to the rest of your body, which causes you to feel tired and puts you in a stupor. To stay alert, eat slightly smaller meals, and avoid starchy carbs. Too much pasta and white bread can deplete your energy, says Mary Jane Detroyer, RD, based in New York City.

Instead of . . . white potatoes
Try . . . sweet potatoes. More flavorful than the white kind, the orange spud is an antioxidant and fiber powerhouse that keeps skin glowing, fires your immune system, and steadies blood sugar—which helps you resist junk food benders. A medium-size baked sweet potato has 60 fewer calories and an extra gram of fiber compared to the white tubers. Try baking sliced sweet potato wedges drizzled with olive oil at 425 degrees until slightly browned, and then sprinkle with sea salt.

Instead of . . . potato chips
Try . . . popcorn. It may seem like a big bunch of air, but these kernels are actually tiny little fiber machines that keep you really full.
Decode the label . . . One cup of popcorn clocks in at about 30 calories, less than 1 gram of fat, and costs only about 25 cents, so this treat won't break the bank or your diet! Compare that to a measly ounce of potato chips, which has 160 calories and 10 grams of fat. Bonus: Since popcorn's so low in calories, you can munch tons of it without guilt, which may trick your mind into eating less later, since you've already inhaled *sooo* much. Stock up on the plain kernels as opposed to the microwave or already-popped packaged kinds, because many of those brands have added butter and oils, making them a lot higher in calories.

MORE REASONS TO GET POPPING

If you're craving comfort food that won't leave you with snacker's remorse, reach for a bowl of popcorn. Popcorn eaters get a whopping 250 percent more whole grains and about 22 percent more fiber than those who don't eat the fluffy white snack, reports the *Journal of the American Dietetic Association*. Skip the kind that comes in a bucket or a bag, since it is loaded with calories and fat, and air-pop your own. Spritz the popped kernels with a little olive oil and sprinkle with garlic salt, grated Parmesan cheese, cinnamon, or whatever spice topping you're in the mood for.

Instead of . . . ranch dip

Try . . . hummus.

Decode the label . . . While 2 tablespoons of ranch dip has zero fiber and 110 calories, this chickpea spread is packed with protein and 2 grams of fiber—both of which help curb hunger—and has only about 50 calories. Eat hummus with veggies like baby carrots for a crunchy snack to crank up your fiber intake even more.

Instead of . . . pita or tortilla chips

Try . . . whole grain crackers.

Decode the label . . . An ounce of both corn tortilla chips and multigrain pita chips has about 140 calories, 2 grams of fiber or less, and 6 grams of fat. You'll get much more value for your nutritional buck if you go for crispbreads such as Finn Crisps, which have 87 calories, 5.4 grams of fiber, and less than 1 gram of fat per ounce. Another good bet are flatbreads such as Doctor Kracker's, which weigh in at 113 calories, 3.4 grams of fiber, and 4.5 grams of fat.

Instead of . . . sides of pasta or white noodles

Try . . . long-grain or brown rice, quinoa, or beans.

Decode the label . . . A cup of pasta has 2.4 grams of fiber, while egg noodles have less than 2 grams. Here is how higher-fiber alternatives stack up: Brown rice has 3.5 grams, quinoa has 5.2 grams (and is packed with muscle-building protein), and beans can have up to 15 grams! One cup of black beans will give you half of your daily fiber goal for less than 230 calories, so try eating them as a side or adding them to salads and soups.

WHAT KIND OF CARBS SHOULD I EAT?

With all the hype about good versus bad carbs, it can be confusing to know which type is which. The good carbs are typically high in fiber to help with your digestion, and there are two types of fiber, soluble and insoluble, which act in different ways to benefit your diet.

You may have heard your grandma refer to insoluble fiber as roughage, because it doesn't dissolve in water and bulks up your stool to sweep out unhealthy or undigestible foods. Since your body has to work to move it through your digestive tract, it also helps boost metabolism. That means it takes more energy (and calories!) to digest whole grain carbs, such as shredded wheat, than it does white carbs that have the fiber stripped from them when they're processed, such as corn flakes. Whole grain cereals, leafy greens, cruciferous veggies such as cauliflower, and some fruits such as apples are good sources of insoluble fiber.

Soluble fiber does dissolve in water and swells up in your stomach to make you feel full so you're apt to eat fewer calories. Plus, it helps pull cholesterol out of your body. Slow-cooked rolled oats, beans, and fruits such as oranges and pears are all packed with the soluble kind.

No matter the type of fiber, it won't get digested before you get rid of it by, well, going to the bathroom, so it doesn't pack any calories. That's why when you look at a food label, you can subtract the grams of fiber from the total carbohydrates to figure out the net carbs—or carbs that will add to your calorie count. For example, if the nutrition label for a slice of bread says it has 21 grams of carbohydrates and 7 grams of fiber, you can subtract 7 from 21 to find out that that slice has only 14 grams of net carbohydrates. So you can eat as many carbohydrates in the form of fiber as you want, but should get no more than 200 grams of net carbohydrates a day. Also scour food labels for whole grains in the ingredient list, such as whole oats, whole wheat, and whole rye.

BIKINI DIET MEAL PLAN WEEK 6

Turn to the Month 2 Bikini Diet Meal Plan Cheat Sheet on page 72 for a quick overview on what to eat this week, or go to Chapter 14, page 170, for details on portion sizes and recipes. This week is all about fitting in more of the F word—fiber. You don't have to stress about how to fit in 30 grams of fiber a day, because we've done the math for you. Simply follow this week's meal plan and you'll reach your goal, no number-crunching required. And if you want experiment with other fiber-filled options for a little more variety, check out the below suggested swaps for meals.

Day 1

Try to fit in a serving of fiber-packed Brussels sprouts by swapping 'em in for snow peas with your Macadamia-Crusted Tilapia Fillet with Pineapple Salsa dinner entrée tonight.

Day 4

Opt to have a side of ½ cup of black beans instead of the suggested baked sweet potato with your Tropical Mahi Mahi Salad to fill up on a different kind of protein-packed fiber.

Day 5

Try seeing if you fill up faster by starting today's lunch with a bowl of veggie broth–based (not cream-based!) soup in place of the apple before you eat the Thai Chopped Chicken Salad.

HOT & HEALTHY WORKOUT WEEK 6

Here's what to do this week:

◆ Morning Cardio Blast, 4 to 5 times this week, as soon as you wake up (See page 209.)
◆ Barry's Bootcamp Rubber Band Workout, twice a week—but not on consecutive days! (See page 209.)
◆ Tracy Anderson's Lower-Body Blast, twice this week—but not on consecutive days! (See page 210.)

◆ Feel-Good Fitness day once this week (See page 211.)
◆ Rest and recover—2 days this week, but not on consecutive days!

Like Brazilian bikini bottoms? Tracy Anderson's Lower-Body Blast delivers leaner legs, a firmer bum, and A-list abs. Be sure to use a sturdy chair on an even surface, so you don't bail. You'll engage your core muscles as you work to balance throughout each move. The result: sexy, show-off abs.

Keep going with your lighter resistance bands this week, but make sure it doesn't feel too easy, or you won't keep seeing results. "Remember to keep the *work* in *work*out," says Barry Jay of Barry's Bootcamp. "Keep pushing yourself to do more reps or use a heavier band if you're feeling good, but never sacrifice form while using resistance bands to make the sculpting moves most effective."

(UN)GUILTY PLEASURE: TREAT YOURSELF TO SEXY WORKOUT GEAR

Wearing workout gear that you actually feel good in—as opposed to those baggy old sweats—boosts your motivation to hit the gym. Reward yourself for making it to the halfway mark of the program—and motivate yourself to keep going—by updating your exercise wardrobe with these picks that are so cute you won't be able to wait to slip into them and get moving.

The Active Bag (activyst.com)

This brand-new turquoise or coral waterproof bag has separate compartments for shoes, sweaty clothes, yoga mats, and even your laptop. It fits all your stuff without being bulky and is cute enough to take both to the gym and away for a weekend beach trip. Bonus: Proceeds from sales help girls in need play sports.

SOUNDING OFF!

Maria Sharapova, your unladylike on-court noises have been officially vindicated. Grunting before a strength move increases power by 7 percent, a study by researchers at Iowa State University reported. You don't have to go all cavewoman at the gym, but the occasional yelp could help you eke out a few more reps.

Jubralee Bra (movingcomfort.com)

No need to accept the pancake boob fate when looking for a sports bra that keeps your breasts from bouncing: The Jubralee both encapsulates and elevates breasts for a flattering shape while cutting breast acceleration in half.

Power Y Tank Luon Light (shop.lululemon.com)

The built-in shelf bra has removable pads for added coverage and the soft, racer-back straps don't dig in or make you feel restricted when you're doing yoga twists and heart openers. The tank is long enough that it won't ride up.

Women's Urban Gym Tee (movingcomfort.com)

Perfect for Zumba, dance, or any other gym class, this trendy tee has dolman sleeves and ribbon accents. Plus, it's green: It's made with recycled coffee grounds for moisture management and odor control.

890v3 Women's Sneaker (newbalance.com)

These kicks will make you feel light on your feet, thanks to the special REVlite foam that's 30 percent lighter than traditional foams but just as durable. The heel is also dropped slightly to bring the sole closer to the ground for better stability—whether you're logging miles on the treadmill or doing weighted lunges.

Power Walk 603 Sneakers (prospecs-usa.com)

New to the United States from Korea, these shoes are for serious power walkers. Their midsole's technology gives stability to hold your foot supersecure and keep your feet/ankles and hips lined up properly. Plus, the deep purple shoes with neon yellow laces and mesh accents look cool enough to wear walking around town with your favorite T-shirt and jeans.

PINK Timex Marathon GPS (amazon.com)

Sticking to your same old walking or running route gets boring, yet you may not want to veer off the beaten path because you won't know how many miles you're logging. This pink watch tracks distance, time, and even calories burned to take the guesswork out of exercise. It motivates you to keep going because it helps you track your progress.

Skirt Sports Gym Girl Ultra Skirt (skirtsports.com/stores)

While many exercise shorts tend to be shapeless or ride up, this sports skirt has built-in shorties made of compression mesh to keep them in place. Plus, they're pretty enough to wear from the gym to meet a friend for coffee. Two hidden pockets inside can fit essentials such as an energy bar, keys, or iPod. You can even weave the cord through a little music port on the skirt to rock out while you work out.

SUCCESS TRACKER:

Bikini Body Checklist Week 6

☐ I met my goal of eating 30 grams of fiber a day by following the weekly meal plan.

☐ I swapped out low-fiber, refined carbs like potato chips and white breads for high-quality carbs, such as popcorn and whole grain breads.

☐ I've fit more veggies into my daily diet.

☐ I've followed the Bikini Diet meal plan.

☐ I've followed the Hot & Healthy Workout plan.

☐ I've treated myself to at least one cute new workout item or outfit as a reward for making it halfway through the Cosmo Bikini Diet so I feel confident and sexy when I'm at the gym.

Week 6 Measurements

Weight _____

Waist _____

Chest _____

Hips _____

This week I feel _____

_____

_____

_____

_____

_____

_____

_____

_____

_____

CHAPTER SEVEN

HEALTHY FAT IS YOUR FRIEND

WEEK #7

THE LOWDOWN Does the following eating routine sound at all familiar? You have low-fat yogurt for breakfast; a fat-free microwave meal for lunch; and a big salad topped with fat-free chicken breast and fat-free dressing for dinner.

You've been so "good" that you even treat yourself to a cup of low-fat fro-yo for dessert. While you may think you're eating healthy, avoiding fat like an ex-boyfriend you regret can actually be bikini body sabotage. This chapter includes:

◆ The secret of how eating fat can actually help slim your waist
◆ The best foods for fitting more "good fats" into your diet
◆ Easy ways to use those ingredients in your meals and snacks
◆ Fun, simple tricks to move more all day long to really rev your weight loss
◆ Why laughing is good for your mood *and* body

7 WAYS HEALTHY FAT DOES A BIKINI BODY GOOD

Like calories, all fat is not created equal. The "bad" guys are saturated fats (which boost cholesterol and heart disease risk) and trans fats (some are naturally occurring, but most come from unsaturated fats that have been chemically morphed and put in processed foods such as cakes, doughnuts, and French fries to up their shelf lives).

The "good" guys, on the other hand, are unsaturated fats. A trick to remember which type is the healthy kind might be to tell yourself that this week's (*un*)diet secret is to eat more *un*saturated fats. The good kinds include belly-fat-fighting monounsaturated fats (aka MUFAs), and polyunsaturated fats (one type is immune-boosting omega-3 fatty acids). Here are the top reasons why fitting more unsaturated fats into your diet is so good for your bikini body.

1 **It melts belly fat.** When it comes to boosting your metabolism, a diet high in healthy fats may trump a low-fat diet—so long as you time your meals correctly. Researchers from the Hebrew University of Jerusalem discovered that a scheduled high-fat diet actually helped mice burn *more* fat rather than storing that fat around their middles. The key to rewiring your metabolism may be to eat healthy fat on an empty stomach (in the morning after fasting all night or during your afternoon slump rather than eating something fatty following a big meal) so that fat gets used as energy rather than stored around your waist.

2 **It makes food taste good.** Eating is one of life's greatest pleasures, and fat gives food a major flavor boost. Think about how much buzz the Mediterranean diet has gotten for being both delicious and healthy. This eating style uses plenty of healthy, monounsaturated fat–packed olive oil for dipping fresh-baked bread and sautéing fish and lean meat. Yum!

3 **It keeps you happy.** If you're eating mostly fat-free foods, you could be prone to major mood swings. Diets with less than 25 percent of calories from fat have been linked to increased anxiety, according to a study in the *British Journal of Nutrition*. Other research finds that depriving your brain of omega-3s could be a depression culprit, since more than half of your brain mass is made up of healthy fats. The good news is that eating more omega-3s can boost mood: Studies show that having omega-3-rich seafood two or more times a week may slash your odds of the blues by 50 percent.

4 **It helps you absorb vitamins and nutrients.** Going fat free can make you nutrient deficient. That's because your body won't be able to use fat-soluble vitamins—A, K, D, and E—if you don't eat fat! It's a smart idea to top your green leafy salads with small amounts of foods that have healthy fat, such as slivered almonds, olive-oil-based dressings, or sliced avocadoes, to help your body better absorb vitamins.

5 **It protects your heart.** Swapping saturated fats, like the kind in butter, for healthier unsaturated fats, like the kind in canola or olive oil, may slash your risk of heart disease by *almost 20 percent*, according to a study in the journal *PLoS Medicine*. Plus, mono- and polyunsaturated fats have been linked with lowering LDL, or "bad" cholesterol, and raising HDL, or "good" cholesterol. Try swapping heart-healthy olive oil for butter on toast and when cooking eggs. There are plenty of expensive brands, but pretty much any cold-pressed extra-virgin olive oil that you buy will give you the same nutrients.

6 **It prettifies your complexion.** Fatty acids hydrate your skin cells plus give your skin a lit-from-within luminosity. How? They help build and strengthen cell membranes to allow water and nutrients in and keep toxins out.

SPRITZ ON OIL

Sure, olive, canola, and soybean oils are packed with healthy fats and add flavor, but the secret to maxing out their benefits and slimming your waistline is to go light-handed. A serving of oil is only 1 tablespoon—about the size of a water bottle cap—and has 119 calories. Pouring on oil to sauté fish and vegetables or oil-based dressings over your salads means you could easily eat 4 tablespoons' worth in one meal—almost 480 calories in oil alone! For a no-sweat way to go easy, try putting oil in a spray bottle and spritzing on rather than pouring. You'll get all the health benefits while saving yourself hundreds of calories.

7 **It fills you up.** Fat doesn't spike blood sugar levels and can take up to 6 hours to fully digest (more time than starches or even protein). Fats help to keep you full longer, because each gram of fat has 9 calories (compared to carbs and protein, which only have 4 calories per gram). The result? It takes your body longer to digest them to ward off an afternoon snack attack.

STOCK YOUR KITCHEN WITH THESE HEALTHY-FAT FOODS

AVOCADOS Though they taste like a vegetable, avocados are technically fruits—and are high in heart-healthy fats. Their creamy texture and mild, nutty flavor make them a great swap for butter or mayonnaise on sandwiches. Or make a healthier dip for your next girls' night by mashing together a medium avocado with chopped tomatoes, a clove or two of diced garlic, a squeeze of lime juice, and salt and pepper to taste for homemade guacamole.

FATTY FISH Some fish are loaded with omega-3 fatty acids, including salmon, mackerel, herring, tuna, and sardines. The American Heart Association recommends having at least two servings of fish per week—just like our Bikini Diet!

NUT BUTTERS A great source of unsaturated fat, nut butters make great breakfast spreads. Try a tablespoon of peanut, almond, or cashew butter on your whole wheat toast or English muffin.

NUTS All nuts deliver healthy fats, including almonds, Brazil nuts, cashews, chestnuts, hazelnuts, macadamia nuts, peanuts, pecans, pine nuts, pistachios, and walnuts. Add chopped walnuts to your yogurt in the morning, or to refuel during an afternoon slump, replace low-fat snacks like granola bars with an ounce of mixed nuts.

OILS Safflower, olive, flaxseed, canola, sunflower, grapeseed, soybean, and many other types of oils have healthy fats. At dinner, splash olive oil with balsamic vinegar on your side salad instead of low-fat dressing, or try stirring flaxseed oil into your a.m. smoothie.

SEEDS Pumpkin, flaxseed, sunflower, and other seeds are a tasty, crunchy way to add healthy fats to your diet, and they're easy to use in moderation. Sprinkle them over cereal and salads or add a small handful to your trail mix. Fun fact: Chia seeds, which come from South America but made their North American debut in the '80s with the Chia Pet, are actually the highest natural plant source of omega-3s. Try mixing chia seeds in your oatmeal or smoothie for an omega-3-packed breakfast.

BIKINI DIET MEAL PLAN WEEK 7

Turn to the Month 2 Bikini Diet Meal Plan Cheat Sheet on page 72 for a quick overview on what to eat this week, or go to Chapter 14, page 170, for details on portion sizes and recipes. If you've been following the Cosmo Bikini Diet meal plans, you've been filling up on healthy fats for the past 6 weeks. In fact, about 30 percent of your daily calories are coming from fats, and they're mostly all the beautifying, good-for-you kind! If you've noticed that you're feeling hunger pangs less often, and have glossier hair and brighter skin, you can probably thank all those unsaturated fats you've been noshing.

HOT & HEALTHY WORKOUT WEEK 7

Here's what to do this week:

◆ Morning Cardio Blast, 4 to 5 times this week, as soon as you wake up (See page 212.)
◆ Barry's Bootcamp Rubber Band Workout, twice this week—but not on consecutive days! (See page 212.)
◆ Tracy Anderson's Get a Tight, Sexy Core toning routine, twice this week—but not on consecutive days! (See page 213.)
◆ Feel-Good Fitness day once this week (See page 214.)
◆ Rest and recover—2 days this week, but not on consecutive days!

Tracy Anderson's Get a Tight, Sexy Core sessions will help sculpt that six-pack, as you're in prime belly-fat-melting mode at this point in the diet. Her easy moves tone your abs, obliques, and waist all at the same time, so you'll be bikini ready ASAP.

Since you've been using your lighter band for the past 2 weeks, it's time to graduate to the thicker, heavier resistance band for your workouts this week to force your muscles to work harder. Be sure to really focus on the muscles that you're working during Barry's Bootcamp Rubber Band Workout. By paying attention to the specific muscles you're toning, you'll be able to have better form, which makes for even more defined results. "For example, when doing a bicep curl, we always ask our clients to 'put your brain in the muscle you're working' in order to minimize using your other muscles to compensate, such as your back or shoulders," says Barry Jay of Barry's Bootcamp.

Take a Stand to Burn Fat and Slim Down

You drive to the office. Take the elevator to your floor. Camp out in front of your computer for 8 hours. Hit the gym after work. Crash on your couch catching up on *Girls* reruns. Rinse. Repeat.

Sure, you may have fit in a workout (which helps you get toned), but spending the rest of the day on your butt will keep you from getting your sexiest bikini body. That's because it's those little moves you make all throughout the day that can add up to big weight loss. In fact, people who move more all day long (think: pacing while chatting on the phone versus staying slumped at your desk) boost their metabolism and burn up to 350 extra calories a day, according to researchers at the Mayo Clinic in Rochester, Minnesota. That extra 350 calories equals almost 37 pounds a year!

Sitting too much not only wreaks havoc on your waistline, it may also be the new smoking: Having your butt planted in a chair for 6 or more hours a day ups your odds of everything from cancer to heart disease to diabetes to early death—for real! And while fitting in exercise by following our easy Hot & Healthy Workout Plan is vital for toning up, even making time to exercise for an hour a day can't completely reverse the life-shortening damage of a (mostly) sedentary lifestyle. So while spending hours on the treadmill won't transform your bod into a lean, mean, fat-burning machine, doing the opposite and staying seated on the couch or at your desk for all of your waking hours outside of your daily workouts could do a number on your health (that's another reason why fitting in 15 minutes of cardio intervals on most days, as well as experimenting with Feel-Good Fitness days that remind you how to enjoy moving your body, are so important). The key is simply to move more all throughout the day—not only when you're working out.

Although you probably can't afford to spend less time studying in the library or to quit your day job, you *can* take a stand to boost blood flow and metabolism, burn calories, and increase energy. Here are some simple ways to move more all day long:

◆ **Stand up for your bikini bod.** You can burn up to an extra 500 calories a day without doing a lot of activity simply by standing rather than sitting. If you can't get away from your desk, try standing to make a phone call or when reading a report.

◆ **Clean house.** Instead of having a movie marathon on the weekend, spend 2 hours getting organized by cleaning out your closets or vacuuming and dusting the house to slash about 408 calories.

◆ **Have a dance-a-thon.** Go out with your girls and move to some live music, or blast your favorite tunes and dance around your living room. Rocking out like this for an hour torches 445 calories—and you'll be having fun, so it won't feel like exercise.

◆ **Pedal away.** Biking is great cardio—plus you have to engage your core muscles to stay balanced. One hour of biking at an easy pace blasts 272 calories—pedal just twice a week, and that's more than 6 pounds dropped in a year. If biking to work or school is an option, try ditching your car a few times a week. To find a bike trail near you, check out TrailLink.com.

◆ **Run some errands.** Spend an evening food shopping and unloading groceries to burn close to 500 calories. Cook dinner to burn 90 more.

◆ **Move on your lunch hour.** A brisk 15-minute walk burns about 100 calories, and it gives you less time to steal a slice of pizza from the box that your cubicle mate ordered for lunch. Or try wearing a pedometer to measure out 10,000 steps a day, or about 5 miles—you'll automatically burn 500 calories without even hitting the gym.

◆ **Take a commercial break.** Even getting off your couch to squeeze in 5 minutes of push-ups or jumping jacks can burn another 50 calories. There may be as many as 10 minutes of commercials during a sitcom, so take 10 to jog in place and burn 91 calories, lift weights to burn 34 calories, or jump rope to burn 113 more.

(UN)GUILTY PLEASURE: GET A DAILY DOSE OF LAUGHTER

Laughing burns calories (15 minutes of chuckling erases the amount in two Hershey's Kisses) and may help keep your blood sugar in check. Volunteers who watched a funny flick reaped about two times lower blood sugar levels compared to when they saw a boring lecture, discovered researchers from the University of Tsukuba in Japan. Experts aren't sure how laughter helps exactly, but speculate giggle fests work tummy muscles to process glucose faster (stable blood sugar levels control appetite).

The best reason to get a daily dose of laughter is that it makes you feel good and busts stress. Put your funniest pal on speed dial to get your daily fix, or check out FunnyorDie.com for hysterical videos, pictures, and jokes.

SUCCESS TRACKER:

Bikini Body Checklist Week 7

☐ I've stocked my kitchen with healthy-fat foods, and have made a serious effort to use them in moderation in all of my meals and snacks.

☐ I've found small ways to move more all day long, like pacing while I talk on the phone.

☐ I've followed the Bikini Diet meal plan.

☐ I've followed the Hot & Healthy Workout plan.

☐ I've gotten a daily dose of laughter.

Week 7 Measurements

Weight_____

Waist_____

Chest_____

Hips_____

This week I feel _____

_____

_____

_____

_____

_____

_____

_____

_____

_____

_____

_____

_____

_____

CHAPTER EIGHT

UP YOUR PROTEIN POWER

WEEK #8

THE LOWDOWN By now you've learned a ton of new healthy-eating secrets and have made fitting in fitness a habit. You're also officially two-thirds of the way to your best bikini body ever.

You've discovered that it's not only the *number* of calories you consume but also the *type* that counts when it comes to slimming down. This week's slim-down secret weapon is learning why and how to fill up on protein, an important nutritional component of the Bikini Diet meal plans.

Plus, you'll find out if there really is a best time to exercise; get Jillian Michaels's exercise motivation trick; and discover ways to turn off your brain so you can chill out—no matter how hectic life gets.

PROTEIN: THE WEIGHT-LOSS WONDER

Research has found that having more protein keeps you feeling full longer, so you can eat less food overall and still feel satisfied. A recent study backs up this theory: Researchers from the University of Sydney found that people who ate a diet of 10 percent protein reported feeling hungrier and ate more calories throughout the day—mostly from mindless snacking—than those eating a 15 percent protein diet. Researchers estimated that the extra calories consumed by participants on the lower-protein diet could add up to an extra 2.2 pounds of weight gain *a month*.

Protein also helps your body build and maintain lean muscle, and muscles burn calories, even when you're resting, for a metabolic boost. Plus, lean muscle transforms your body by making you look more firm and toned (and who wants thigh jiggle on the beach?).

To make sure you have plenty of protein power, the Cosmo Bikini Diet meal plans all average about 20 percent of daily calories from protein (which range from 1,600 to 1,650, including the Flex Calories), or about 80 grams.

If you're a granola bar or bagel type of girl, try giving your breakfast a protein makeover. Adding protein to your morning meal might be the ultimate appetite suppressor—and that's why our Cosmo Bikini Diet breakfasts are protein packed. People who eat higher amounts of protein at breakfast feel more satisfied and are less likely to reach for unhealthy snacks later on as compared to those who skimp on protein in the a.m., according to the journal *Obesity*. In fact, eating a high-protein breakfast may keep you from eating an extra 200 calories during nighttime snacking (or about as many calories as you burned doing your 15 minutes of morning cardio).

Rather than obsessively counting every gram of protein you eat, you can make some easy switches that up your protein intake without upping your overall calories. Here are some no-sweat swaps to sneak in more protein:

Instead of . . . ½ cup granola with 1 cup berries (7 g protein, 250 calories)
Try . . . ½ cup low-fat cottage cheese with 1 cup berries (15 g protein, 131 calories)

Instead of . . . 6-inch pancake sans butter or syrup (5 g protein, 175 calories)
Try . . . 1 cup low-fat plain yogurt with ½ cup apricots
(13 g protein, 183 calories)

Instead of . . . 1 ¼ cups mashed potatoes (5 g protein, 296 calories)
Try . . . 1 ¼ cups vegetarian baked beans (15 g protein, 295 calories)
Tip: Go for the no-sugar added kind to cut back on unnecessary sugar.

Instead of . . . 1 cup cooked spaghetti, no sauce (7 g protein, 197 calories)
Try . . . ¾ cup cooked brown lentils flavored with Italian seasoning and diced cooked carrots (14 g protein, 173 calories)

YOUR PROTEIN GUIDE

The key to this week's diet secret is that every snack or meal you eat has some type of lean protein (think: flank steak, white fish, tofu, beans, low-fat cheese). You've been eating lean proteins with every meal for a few weeks now if you've been following the weekly meal plans, so you're already on track!

Here's the lowdown on how many grams of protein are packed into different foods, so you can mix and match them into your meals and snacks to keep from getting stuck in a rut once you've completed the Cosmo Bikini Diet. Again, don't stress about counting grams of protein, but just use them as general guidelines for adding more protein picks to your meals and snacks.

Beans

Legumes help with weight loss double-time because they score big on both filling protein and fiber. Try swapping meat for beans in one or two of your meals to fit in more fiber without skimping on protein. Here is how much a cup contains:

Black beans, 15 g
Chickpeas, 15 g
Kidney beans, 15 g
Lentils, 16 g
Peas, 8 g

Dairy & Eggs

Enjoying low-fat dairy like yogurt and milk may help melt flab. Research has found dieters who ate three to four servings of calcium-rich dairy a day could eat 150 to 200 *more* overall calories while still losing weight as compared to dieters eating only two servings a day or less, according to the University of Tennessee. Other studies find people who are low on calcium have higher levels of body fat. Here is how popular dairy picks bank in the protein department. (A serving of cheese is 1 ounce, milk is 1 cup, and yogurt is 6 ounces.)

Cheddar cheese, 7 g
Cream cheese, 2 g
Feta cheese, 4 g
Goat cheese, 6 g
Greek yogurt, 16 g
Low-fat cottage cheese, 28 g
Mozzarella cheese (part skim), 7 g
One large egg, 6 g
Parmesan cheese, 11 g
Provolone cheese, 7 g
Regular yogurt, 7 g
Ricotta cheese (part skim), 3 g
Swiss cheese, 8 g
Whole or fat-free milk, 8 g

Fish

Go for these kinds of swimmers that are low in toxic mercury. (Look for low-mercury brands of canned tuna, such as Fishing Vessel St. Jude.) Bonus: Most are also high in omega-3s, a type of fatty acid linked with lower levels of depression, less painful periods, and reduced risk of heart disease. A 4-ounce serving of the following has:

Canned tuna, 20 g
Cod, 26 g
Halibut, 30 g
Mahi mahi, 32 g
Sardines, 23 g
Scallops, 20 g
Shrimp, 18 g
Trout, 30 g
Wild salmon, 35 g

Lean Meat

Just as all calories are not created equal, neither are all proteins. In fact, the type of protein you eat matters because lean proteins like grilled chicken have been linked to more weight loss and better health as compared to marbled, fattier types like rib-eye steak. Here is how much protein is packed in a typical 4-ounce serving of lean meat.

Boneless cured ham, 25 g
Boneless top loin pork chop, 25 g
Flank steak, 32 g
Lean veal loin, 38 g
Ground beef (95% lean), 33 g
Skinless chicken breast, 27 g
Skinless turkey breast, 34 g

Nuts & Seeds

You may have sworn off nuts and seeds because they're high in calories and fat, but nuts and seeds are also an appetite suppressant high in protein, fiber, and healthy fats. In fact, research shows that people who eat a small portion of nuts two or more times a week are less likely to gain weight than those who skip nuts, according to the journal *Obesity*. Other studies found that people noshing a handful of nuts a day have higher levels of the happiness hormone serotonin, which is also linked to lower appetite. A portion is a handful or about the size of a shot glass. Here are the protein counts for around 150 to 200 calories per 1-ounce serving (or 2 tablespoons for the nut butters) of the following:

Almonds, 6 g
Almond butter (2 tablespoons), 5 g
Cashews, 4 g
Flaxseeds, 5 g
Peanuts, 7 g
Peanut butter (2 tablespoons), 8 g
Pecans, 3 g
Pistachios, 6 g
Pumpkin seeds, 9 g
Sunflower seeds, 6 g
Walnuts, 4 g

Soy

Unprocessed soy like edamame and tofu may cut your breast cancer risk in half. Here is how to get your soy protein au naturel. One cup of the following has:

Edamame, 17 g
Miso soup, 8 g
Tofu, 10 g

Q: IS THERE A BEST TIME TO EXERCISE?

A: Yes. Whenever you want! Any workout is a win, and every time offers health perks.

Early Morning Morning exercisers are most likely to fit in a workout, because they get it done before work/friends/life get in the way, according to Cedric Bryant, PhD, chief science officer of the American Council on Exercise.

Midmorning A midmorning workout sets you up to eat a healthy lunch: Exercise curbs your body's production of the hunger-stoking hormone ghrelin.

Lunchtime Working out pumps extra blood to the brain, bathing neurons in oxygen and nutrients. It also stimulates the production of chemicals and hormones that improve concentration and reasoning skills. What 3 o'clock slump?

Afternoon Exercising in the afternoon may help optimize your circadian rhythms, helping you sleep more soundly at night, according to a recent study in the *Journal of Physiology*.

Evening Your body temperature is at its highest in the late afternoon, making your muscles more flexible. Exercise starts to feel easier. Plus, testosterone peaks at this time of day, boosting your strength-training results.

Late Night Although an intense workout late at night can make it tough to fall asleep, doing calming exercise like gentle yoga or tai chi before bed will lower cortisol levels, which will reduce anxiety and make it easier for you to drift off to sleep, according to a Harvard University study.

BIKINI DIET MEAL PLAN WEEK 8

Turn to the Month 2 Bikini Diet Meal Plan Cheat Sheet on page 72 for a quick overview on what to eat this week, or go to Chapter 14, page 170, for details on portion sizes and recipes. You've been filling up on satiating and muscle-building protein for weeks, since you've been following the Cosmo Bikini Diet meal plans. You've learned what to look for when eating out or when you can't follow the plan strictly; for example, lean protein like grilled skinless chicken breasts over fattier cuts such as legs, and high-fiber plant protein sources like black beans. Keep following the Month 2 Meal Plan and you'll continue to get the right amount of protein to help fuel your muscles and metabolism.

To switch up your protein variety this week, try swapping out your go-to nuts, such as almonds, for a different variety, such as walnuts, cashews, or pecans, for the snack and meal suggestions (just stick to 1-ounce portions no matter the type you're noshing on). Also try switching around your sides, like adding lentils in place of couscous. You could sub a lunch side or snack, such as an apple, with ½ cup of dry-roasted edamame for a crunchy, protein-packed alternative.

HOT & HEALTHY WORKOUT WEEK 8

This is your very last week in the second month of the Cosmo Bikini Diet, and you've no doubt noticed that you're getting tighter and more toned all over. Look back at your measurements from the first week before you started the program and compare them to where you are now for inspiration during your sweat sessions.

Here's what to do this week:

◆ Morning Cardio Blast, 4 to 5 times this week, as soon as you wake up (See page 215.)
◆ Barry's Bootcamp Rubber Band Workout, twice this week—but not on consecutive days! (See page 215.)
◆ Tracy Anderson's Shape Sexy Abs, Superfast! toning routine, twice this week—but not on consecutive days! (See page 216.)
◆ Feel-Good Fitness day once this week (See page 217.)
◆ Rest and recover—2 days this week, but not on consecutive days!

We'll keep the focus on your tummy with Tracy Anderson's Shape Sexy Abs, Superfast! routine. This belly-flattening workout is the next best thing to invisible Spanx (will someone please invent that?). Then you'll stick with the heavier resistance band again this week for your total-body workout.

(UN)GUILTY PLEASURE: CHILL OUT WITH A MEDITATION STYLE THAT MATCHES YOUR PERSONALITY

You've no doubt heard about meditation's mind and body benefits: Stress relief, improved memory, less anxiety, and even better blood sugar have all been linked to channeling some inner peace. But maybe your blood pressure rises just thinking about sitting in lotus position and doing nothing but focusing on your breath, so finding a technique that better suits your personality might be a better way for you to start.

"Everyone can meditate," says Sarah McLean, a meditation teacher based in Sedona, Arizona, and author of *Soul Centered: Transform Your Life in 8 Weeks With Meditation*. "Any activity can become a meditative experience if you're really present in the moment and engage your senses. Simply slowing down and being mindful of what's happening right now—rather than thinking about what you ate yesterday or what you're doing tonight—calms your nervous system."

It may sound silly, but learning to sit still or to simply focus on the here and now for just a few minutes a day can make you happier and more in tune with your emotions and your body. This week try doing 5 minutes a day of any type of meditation—even if it means just letting your mind zone out on your train ride to work. We already talked about how an eating meditation can help you eat less, but here are three more ways to meditate, depending on your interests and passions.

If you're artsy, light a fire. If you're a visual type, try focusing your eyes on a candle flame to help you stay in the moment. Whatever your focus is, continue to bring your attention back (be it to your breath or a flame) every time you notice your attention drift away. Just don't give up! You will have thoughts, because that is what the mind does: It thinks. Stick with it and you'll eventually train your mind to quiet down. Sit about 3 feet from a flame (think: a lit candle or even a crackling fire in the fireplace) at eye level; watch it closely for 5 to 10 minutes; feel any tension slowly melt away.

If you're outdoorsy, take a hike. Try walking for 10 minutes sans iPod. As you stride (no rushing!), stare at the ground about 3 feet in front of you. Notice the sound of your breath, of the birds in the trees, of leaves rustling in the wind. Note the smell of snow or rain in the air. Feel the cool breeze in your hair and focus on the texture of the ground or shadows in front of you. It will be a real challenge at first if you're used to walking and talking on your cell or texting during every little bit of downtime, but learning to be more present will help you enjoy your moments more than if you're always distracted by doing a bunch of different things.

If you're a word lover, find a mantra. Sometimes your mind just needs a place to rest, so repeating calming words in your head can offer stress relief by focusing your brain on a single uplifting thought when it's running on overdrive. To try it, find a quiet place, and sit with your back straight but not rigid. Set a timer for 10 to 15 minutes, and repeat words that will help calm—rather than stimulate—your mind. Try saying "peace" on an inhale and "let go" on your exhale, focusing on the sound of your voice. This helps interrupt your thought process. Practice it often enough and you'll learn to control your mind and any runaway inner dialogue on demand.

SUCCESS TRACKER:

Bikini Body Checklist Week 8

☐ I'm snacking on high-protein foods like seeds and nuts and low-fat dairy.

☐ I've followed the Bikini Diet meal plan so that 20 percent of my daily calories are made up of muscle-building protein.

☐ I've followed the Hot & Healthy Workout plan.

☐ I've practiced settling my mind by doing some kind of meditation for at least 5 minutes every day this week.

Week 8 Measurements

Weight _____

Waist _____

Chest _____

Hips _____

This week I feel _____

_____

_____

_____

_____

_____

_____

_____

_____

_____

_____

_____

_____

_____

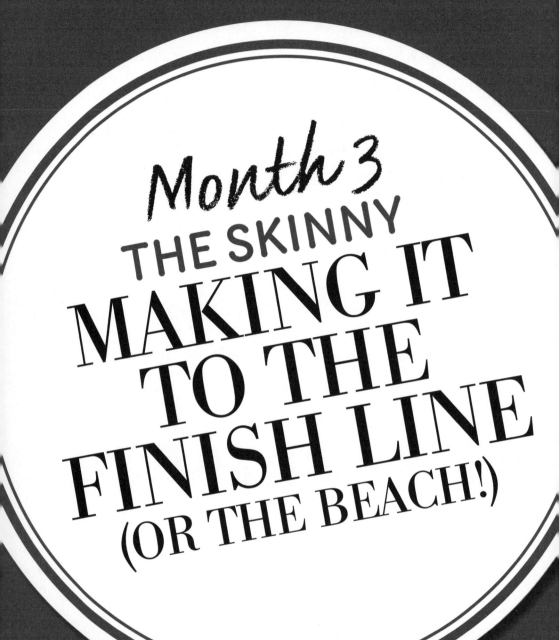

Month 3
THE SKINNY
MAKING IT TO THE FINISH LINE
(OR THE BEACH!)

HEY THERE, SEXY! You've been fueling yourself with nourishing meals, taking care of your body, getting a move on with the weekly Bikini Diet fitness plans, and been making more time to fit in moments of joy with the frequent (Un)Guilty Pleasures. Now that you're near the end of the diet, renew your commitment to getting your strongest, healthiest bikini body by looking back at your goals list and measurements from the beginning to see how far you've come. Then give this last month your all! You'll be sitting with your toes in the sand and a taut tummy soaking up the sun in no time.

THE COSMO BIKINI DIET MEAL PLAN WEEKS 9-12

See page 114 to find out what to eat this month to turn your body into a lean, mean, fat-burning machine as you get ready to hit the beach.

HOT & HEALTHY WORKOUT PLAN (WEEKS 9-12)

For your final month of the Cosmo Bikini Diet, the six-minute toning routines from Tracy Anderson hone in on the most common bikini-body trouble spots, such as your butt and stomach, to really rev up your sculpting power.

You'll also be going back to the twice weekly Barry's Bootcamp Total-Body Strength Circuit from weeks 1 to 4—but with a twist. You've no doubt gotten leaner and stronger, so now it's time to push your body and rev up the sculpting power by increasing the amount of time you do the workout as well as upping your weights. So instead of doing the 20-exercise circuit only once like you did in Month One, now you'll be doing the entire circuit twice for a 40-minute workout. Try using 10-pound weights (or 12-pound if you're feeling really diesel) to do the routine. If the workout becomes too much, just drop down to lighter weights whenever you get too tired.

"We've got two challenge-specific goals this month for you! The first is to do the 15-minute Morning Cardio Blast Workouts without stopping or taking only a few breaks," says Barry Jay of Barry's Bootcamp. "The second is to see how many push-ups on your toes you can do in a row—and then increase this number by the end of Month 3!"

Get ready to lift weights and drop pounds! See page 116 for the Hot & Healthy Workout Cheat Sheet.

BIKINI DIET MEAL PLA

day	BREAKFAST	SNACK	LUNCH
1	Warm quinoa, chia, & fruit cereal (p. 177); coffee or tea	Choc-nutty bananas (p. 182)	Mediterranean chopped salad (p. 178); grapes; unsweetened tea
2	Mixed cereal with berries; coffee or tea (p. 177)	Mini fruit & nut bar and an apple (p. 183)	Grilled cheese and tomato sandwich (p. 178); sliced cucumbers and hummus; fruit & water
3	Veggie & egg melt (p. 177); orange; coffee or tea	Chia seed chocolate almond milk (p. 184)	Taco Salad Bowl (p. 179); unsweetened iced tea
4	Greek yogurt & almonds (p. 177)	Banana coconut smoothie (p. 184)	Cobb salad (p. 179) w/ pita bread and seltzer wate
5	Mango smoothie (p. 178) w/ coffee or tea	Egg salad (p. 184)	Mediterranean platter (p. 179); seltzer water
6	Tomato & Cheese Oatmeal (p. 178); coffee or tea	Trail mix popcorn (p. 185)	Breakfast for Lunch! Straw berry-banana parfait (p. 179 pear; seltzer water
7	EARNED DAY ⟶ (p. 34)		

WEEKLY AVERAGE DAILY NUTRITION FACTS: 1500 calories plus 150 Flex Calories for 1650 total; 45 g total fat, 14 g saturated fat, 0 g trans fat, 12 g monounsaturated fat, 5 g polyunsaturated fat, 235 mg cholesterol, 15 mg sodium, 203 g carbohydrates, 32 g fiber,

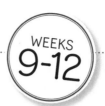
NACK	DINNER	FLEX CALORIES*
it & cheese (p. 182)	Beef burger lettuce wrap (p. 180); crudité and hummus; low-fat milk or milk substitute	Berry cream fro-yo dessert (p. 182) or 150 calories to spend as you like
ack bean & rn salad (p. 183)	Grilled chili-rubbed flank steak (p. 180); baked sweet potato; broccoli; low-fat milk or milk substitute	150 calories to spend as you like
inoa Greek salad 184)	Breakfast for Dinner! Waffles with berries and yogurt (p. 181); orange juice freeze (p. 181)	Grilled coconut crunch pineapple (p. 184) or 150 calories to spend as you like
eese, cucumber & acker sandwiches 184)	Flank steak sandwich (p. 181); roasted asparagus & sweet potato fries (p. 181); w/ unsweetened tea	150 calories to spend as you like
vory spinach bread 184)	Pan-seared tuna w/ lime avocado salsa & roasted butternut squash (p. 181); lemon water	150 calories to spend as you like
etzels & peanut tter (p. 185)	Grilled marinated chicken with grilled zucchini (p. 182); wild rice milk or milk substitute	150 calories to spend as you like

ms sugar, 88 g protein. Ratio of calories
n carbohydrates, protein and fat: 56%
bohydrates, 21% protein and 23% fat.

HOT & HEALTHY
WORKOUT CHEAT SHEET

WEEKS 9-12

You'll find instructions for all the routines in Chapter 15.

DAY	WORKOUT	MINUTES
1	Morning Cardio Blast (pages 219, 222, 225, 228)	15
	Tracy Anderson's Toning Routine (pages 220, 223, 226, 229)	6
	TOTAL WORKOUT TIME	**21**
2	Morning Cardio Blast (pages 219, 222, 225, 228)	15
	Barry's Bootcamp Total-Body Strength Circuit—Times Two! (pages 219, 223, 225, 228)	40
	TOTAL WORKOUT TIME	**55**
3	Rest and recover!	
4	Morning Cardio Blast (pages 219, 222, 225, 228)	15
	Tracy Anderson's Toning Routine (pages 220, 223, 226, 229)	6
	TOTAL WORKOUT TIME	**21**
5	Morning Cardio Blast (pages 219, 222, 225, 228)	15
	Barry's Bootcamp Total-Body Strength Circuit—Times Two! (pages 219, 223, 225, 228)	40
	TOTAL WORKOUT TIME	**55**
6	Rest and recover!	
7	Morning Cardio Blast (Optional) (pages 219, 222, 225, 228)	15
	Feel-Good Fitness day (pages 221, 224, 227, 230)	30-45
	TOTAL WORKOUT TIME	**45-60**

CHAPTER NINE

EAT HEALTHY WHEN EATING OUT

WEEK #9

THE LOWDOWN Sure, it's easy to measure your portions and make good-for-you meal choices when you're cooking at home for yourself, but you also have a life outside your kitchen.

What with weekly happy hours, brunch with the girls, dinner dates, and hitting the party circuit, you're faced with potential calorie-bomb situations every single day. But don't let eating out stress you out: We're here to help you navigate even the most challenging social scenarios so you don't undo all your progress.

The Cosmo Bikini Diet doesn't restrict you from events that involve food. After all, eating and drinking with friends is fun and an important part of your life. The key is to learn the tools that will let you have a good time without sabotaging your waistline.

Think about it: How sexy do you *really* feel after downing a fatty cheeseburger, curly fries, and a few beers when watching the game at a bar? Wouldn't you have just as good a time (and feel a whole lot less bloated) if you went for a grilled chicken sandwich with lettuce, tomato and pickles, and a couple of vodka sodas instead? You may think that sounds lame, but try using the eating-out tricks in this chapter and you'll notice that you feel lighter and more in control of what you put into your mouth, no matter the situation. The even bigger reward will be a slimmer, more toned bikini body that you'll be proud to flaunt at your next pool party.

This week you'll discover the most surprising stay-slim secrets for eating at restaurants, happy hours, parties, and barbecues. Plus, find out how socializing can be good for your waistline, and get ideas on how to throw your own viewing party for your fave TV shows. You'll also kick off the third—and final—workout routine in the Month 3 Bikini Diet Fitness program. Keep your eye on the prize: You're getting close to the finish line!

YOUR BIKINI DIET EATING-OUT SURVIVAL GUIDE

Here's everything you need to know to make smarter food and drink choices when socializing without feeling like you're missing out.

Slim-Down Tricks for Dining at Restaurants

You already know to bring home leftovers of mongo-size restaurant portions. Don't stop there. Slim down any restaurant meal with these surprising strategies.

1 **Scan the menu online.** You're more likely to order a healthy dish if you decide on it in advance rather than if you read mouthwatering menu descriptions on an empty stomach. So before you head to a chain or fast-food restaurant, check out the calorie counts on its website: Subway diners who saw nutrition information before picking out their sandwiches ate fewer calories overall, according to the *American Journal of Public Health.*

For example, instead of having Subway's 6" Chicken and Bacon Ranch Melt for 570 calories and 28 grams of fat, you could go for a 6" Sweet Onion Chicken Terriyaki sub for just 370 calories and 4.5 grams of fat.

2 **Pick a quiet table.** Tucked-away tables can be both intimate *and* slimming: Loud noise and visual distractions (like that overhead TV) can compel you to eat more because you're not focused on how much you're eating.

3 **Be the first to order.** You've decided on grilled salmon, but once you hear your friend's order, you're suddenly dying for steak frites. Speak up first, then shut your menu.

4 **Trade up at brunch.** You don't have to ban brunch with the girls to score a slimmer body. Just remember that making small tweaks to your order can add up to big-time calorie and fat savings. Swap a bagel for an English muffin to slash 220 calories; a whole-milk latte for a skim cappuccino to save 120 calories; and pork sausage for turkey sausage to cut about 125 calories.

5 **Make your lunch skinnier.** Think about little ways to order smarter when out to lunch with coworkers. For your sandwich, you could swap mayo for hummus or mustard and a roll for sliced bread to cut about 200 calories. Go for a salad instead of fries to slash another 300 calories, and you'll save a bikini-busting 500 calories overall (that's about as many calories as you'd burn exercising for an hour!).

6 **Order two appetizers instead of an entrée.** Appetizers are naturally smaller in size, so you can indulge in, say, a crab cake, without risking overdoing it, says Fernando Coppola, executive chef at the W Retreat & Spa in Vieques, Puerto Rico. Ordering two apps instead of a main dish is a no-brainer way to keep portions in check without feeling like you're sapping your willpower by saying no to your fave foods.

7 **Leave something on your plate at dinner.** Leaving a few measly bites of any potato or noodle side dish automatically cuts up to 100 calories because those starches almost always have added butter, oils, or other fats. Skip the risotto dishes altogether if you can—they're usually overloaded with butter and cheese.

8 **Go heavy on the veggies.** Rather than relegating vegetables to a small corner of your plate, make them the star of your meal. You'll fill up on fewer calories by ordering your protein over a bed of steamed or grilled vegetables or salad, recommends Amy Eubanks, executive chef of BLT Fish in New York City. Skip fried appetizers and order a vegetable side dish to help tame your appetite before your main meal comes.

9 **Lean on your server.** It may seem like common sense to look for dishes with bikini-friendly keywords such as *steamed, grilled, poached, broiled,* and *baked* (as compared to *fried, sautéed, loaded, smothered, creamed,* or *crispy*). But healthy eating at a restaurant isn't always so simple.

"Many menus are riddled with fancy, flavor-forward descriptions, and, sadly, most of the dishes are loaded with calories!" says Anthony Bucco, executive chef at The Ryland Inn in Whitehouse Station, New Jersey. "It never hurts to lean on servers for input when selecting your meal, since they should know as well as the chef exactly how the food is prepared. That way, he or she can potentially call out an ingredient that can be easily modified to make your meal healthier." For example, your waiter can tell you that a grilled fish dish is slathered in butter sauce so you can order it without.

10 **Don't empty the baskets.** "The number one diet saboteur is that crusty, warm bread that's placed in front of you before your meal, because most of us don't have the willpower to stop at just one slice and instead eat the entire basket," says Jonathan Rollo, chef and owner of Greenleaf ChopShops in L.A. And that small basket of tortilla chips served at Mexican restaurants often has more calories than your entire meal. Try reminding yourself that you have a big dinner on the way to keep from filling up on empty calories. Or simply ask your waiter to take the basket away to remove the temptation.

11 **Wait to drink until your food arrives.** Downing cocktails to kill time before your meal may up your appetite and block feelings of fullness so you end up eating more, finds researchers from the University of Sussex. Instead, start with a more Bikini Diet–friendly option like soda water with lime or unsweetened iced tea. Drinking healthy, calorie-free liquids help hydrate you and may even take the edge off your hunger.

12 **Savor every bite.** You've no doubt heard of the slow food trend, but what about being a slow eater? "The slower you chew, the easier it is for your body to absorb the nutrients, the more you enjoy your food, and the less you eat overall," says Anthony Fontana, co-owner of Slide restaurant in New York City. Plus, eating slowly gives your body more time to send the "I'm full!" signals to your brain, so you don't overeat.

13 **Customize your salads.** "A lot of restaurants put creative salad items on the menu to entice diners who want to be healthier about their eating choices," says Rollo. "But many of those salads are loaded with cheese, oily dressings, and croutons— and can actually pack a thousand calories into an innocent-looking bowl of greens."

Remember that salads can be made to order and that you can ask for things to be put on the side or excluded. "When it comes to eating out, restaurants are guest hospitality businesses who want to please their customers, so you should be able to manipulate the menu a bit." Try Rollo's tricks for slimming down your salad.

◆ **Don't be cheesy.** "There are very few restaurant salads out there that don't add cheese because it's an easy way to round out the flavors," says Rollo. "You can order it without cheese or ask for it on the side so you can portion it yourself rather than having the line cook do it for you."

◆ **Dress it smart.** "Those reduced-calorie and fat-free dressings are often full of chemicals and added sugars," says Rollo. Instead of ordering lite dressings or heavier ranch kinds, go for vinaigrettes that use fruit as their sweetener for less refined sugar or a tangy balsamic vinaigrette that's likely made with few ingredients or chemicals. "Skipping the dressing and ordering lemon juice and olive oil on the side puts you in control of the amount you use, and is an easy way to cut the volume of dressing in half," says Rollo.

◆ **Skip the croutons.** "Croutons may be delicious, but they're made by taking crusty bread and coating it in oil," says Rollo. "Eating them means you're filling up on saturated fat and added salt." Ask to swap the croutons for, say, chickpeas or dry, roasted nuts for a healthier, protein-packed crunch.

◆ **Make it sweet.** "A lot of times I end up putting chopped fruits into my salads, such as grilled pineapple, apples, peaches, figs, and grapes," says Rollo. "They have natural sugars to add robust flavors, and grilling fruit gives it a smokiness and depth of flavor without adding extra calories and fat."

Slim Down Your Happy Hour

Choosing the right cocktails can save you literally hundreds of empty calories. It might be a good idea, however, to limit yourself to two or three drinks at happy hour, because getting a buzz can:

1. Lower your inhibitions and willpower so you reach for fatty food

2. Trigger cravings

3. Make you more likely to binge eat when you get home from the bar

So go for these skinny drink picks to keep your night out light in calories.
SKIP Energy + Vodka Drink
SIP Vodka Soda
The caffeine in energy drinks keeps you from feeling alcohol's effects, meaning you won't realize how drunk you are. And that will likely make you drink more empty calories (not to mention give you a killer hangover). So ask for calorie-free club soda with your vodka to sidestep caffeine's less-than-ideal side effects.

SKIP Margarita
SIP Tequila, Club Soda, and Lime
When you mix alcohol with something sugary, you're not only consuming extra calories, you also may drink more of it. Tip: Opt to have your drink on the rocks. Ice reduces the volume of liquid in your glass so you'll slash even more calories.

SKIP Chocolate Martini
SIP Regular Martini
Extra ingredients such as crème de cacao and chocolate syrup make this little 2½-ounce drink pack almost 440 calories—and it goes down fast! A traditional martini has only 160 calories, or about one-third less!

SKIP Long Island Iced Tea
SIP Champagne
Those potent Long Island Iced Teas aren't only packed with alcohol—they're also packed with mega calories. You'll sip more than 600 with just one glass, and that's more calories than one of your Bikini Diet dinners! For a classy, refreshing drink that has only about 78 calories, try sipping a glass of bubbly.

SKIP Dark Beer
SIP Lite Beer
As a general rule of thumb, most regular stouts have up to twice as many calories as so-called lite beers. One bottle of Samuel Adam's Boston Lager, for example, has nearly 200 calories compared to Beck's Premier Light's 65 calories. One surprisingly low-calorie dark beer is Guinness, which has only 126 calories in a 12-ounce bottle.

SKIP Sangria
SIP Red Wine
That fruity Spanish punch is filled with 16 grams of sugar in a single glass—and it's usually served in pitchers in restaurants so you rarely drink just one! A smarter bet is to go for a plain old glass of red wine, which is much lower in sugar, to keep your appetite in check so you don't go on a chocolate or chips bender when you get home.

Slim-Down Tricks for a Party
Eat, drink and be merry: There are some great slimming strategies for surviving a party without wrecking your diet.

The first is to **go for foods that make you eat less**. Fill up on any of these four nutrient-packed snacks *before* you go to a party and you'll be too full to stuff yourself silly.

1. HUMMUS This chickpea spread is packed with protein and fiber, both of which help curb hunger. Have 2 tablespoons with veggies or some whole-grain crackers to crank up your fiber intake even more.

2. LOW-FAT GREEK YOGURT Protein takes a long time to leave the stomach, and this dairy wonder contains double the amount found in regular yogurt.

3. VEGETABLE SOUP Remember: Just a cup keeps you full for two reasons: One, veggies are loaded with fiber, which makes you feel satiated for longer, and two, the water-based broth takes up a lot of room in your stomach, leaving less space for snacks.

4. ALMONDS They contain protein, fiber, and good fat, all of which slow down digestion—meaning it takes more time for you to feel hungry again. A little goes a long way: Aim for a small handful (about 14 nuts), which is roughly 100 calories.

The second party-survival strategy is to **go for foods that fuel you** rather than make you feel heavy. We give these three tasty, power-packed party hors d'oeuvres the green light.

1. MOZZARELLA The inevitable cheese tray is tough to ignore. Reach for mozzarella, which has more protein and less fat than most other cheeses.

2. SHRIMP COCKTAIL It's all lean protein, which keeps you alert. But don't overindulge on cocktail sauce—the added sugar has the reverse effect.

3. CRUDITÉS Crunchy veggies, such as carrots, celery, and cauliflower, are not only low-calorie, fiber-filled eats, they can also help brighten your smile by gently scraping away plaque.

NEVER GO TO HAPPY HOUR HUNGRY!

Beware that happy hour falls in that zone between lunch and dinner, so you want to make sure you don't show up starving and overdose on chicken fingers and fries! "Just as you wouldn't think of leaving the house without your keys, get into the habit of packing portable, healthy snacks to tide you over," says Rollo. "Stores like Trader Joe's do a good job of putting together individually-packed snacks, like trail mix and mini carrots, that you can easily toss into your purse."

IS WINE THE NEW DIET DRINK?

Research has found that wine (seriously, wine!) can help keep your weight in check. Drinking it in moderation—that means about a glass a day—has some awesome perks. We asked doctors to explain.

HAPPY HOUR DOES YOUR BODY GOOD...

The evidence is impressive. Researchers kept tabs on nearly 20,000 normal-weight women for 13 years. Over time, the women who drank a glass or two of red wine a day were 30 percent less likely to be overweight than the nondrinkers (they tracked women who drank liquor and beer too, but the link was strongest for red wine). That's not surprising, since vino has other benefits. "It's rich in antioxidants that reduce cholesterol and blood pressure," says Jana Klauer, MD, a New York City physician specializing in nutrition and metabolism.

One reason wine may contribute to a healthy weight is that digesting booze triggers your body to torch calories. "Women make smaller amounts of the enzyme that metabolizes alcohol than men do, so to digest a drink, they have to keep producing it, which requires the body to burn energy," says Dr. Klauer. That means you're likely to see more of a benefit than your guy, since his body doesn't have to work as hard to digest a glass of the grape.

"Alcohol also may burn calories due to a process called thermogenesis," says Lu Wang, MD, PhD, the lead study author and member of the division of preventive medicine at Boston's Brigham and Women's Hospital. Alcohol raises your body temperature (one reason some people get red cheeks when drinking), causing the body to burn calories to create heat.

...BUT THAT'S NOT ALL

The study also showed that women who drank moderately ate less. While researchers can't say why, it's possible that they were more likely to slow down and savor their food and drink.

If you combine all these factors, drinking wine could lead to taking in fewer calories while your body is burning energy, meaning you're less likely to gain weight, says Dr. Wang. Awesome, but you don't want to replace food with wine—you'll miss out on key nutrients and wind up schnockered. And keep in mind that wine has calories: about 125 for 5 ounces. "That's why drinking isn't a weight-loss strategy on its own," says Dr. Klauer. Overdoing it is linked to health risks you don't want to take, like breast cancer. "But having a glass," says Dr. Klauer, "along with a healthy diet and exercise, seems to be a marker for a healthier lifestyle." Hey, we'll *salud* to that.

Slim-down tricks for a barbecue

The fatty cuts of meat, creamy dips, and potato salad taking center stage at most barbecues can all add up to more calories than you bargained for. To slim down your next grill fest without sacrificing flavor, try these seven simple tricks.

1 **Make it a wrap.** Ditch the bun by placing pulled pork or shredded chicken on a large lettuce leaf to save 110 calories. Layer with carrots, tomatoes, cucumbers, and onions, and roll up to eat.

2 **Dip wisely.** Instead of dipping greasy chips in fat-packed sour cream, try serving baked tortilla chips or whole-wheat pita wedges with low-fat refried beans and chunky salsa to eat 109 fewer calories. Bonus: It's a tasty way to sneak in an extra serving of veggies.

3 **Go for leaner meat.** Swap pork sausage for turkey sausage. Or opt for grilled fish, such as tilapia brushed with olive oil and herbs, over fattier cuts of meat like chicken legs. This will save you about 135 to 145 calories so you can sip a brewskie, guilt free.

4 **Be salad savvy.** Take advantage of seasonal produce while slimming your waist: Trade a side of traditional potato salad for sliced tomatoes, cucumbers, and onions tossed with fat-free Italian dressing and you'll save yourself 258 calories.

5 **Swap beef for turkey or chicken burgers.** You'll save one-third the fat and half the calories. "When you make the patties, feel free to mix in robust flavors to blow your guests' minds, such as chopped roasted garlic and shallots, jalapeno, grilled onions, and lots of herbs and spices," says Rollo. "These are practically calorie-free additions, but the flavor boost means you don't need to slather a bunch of sauce or cheese on the burger to make it taste good!"

6 **Grill fruit for dessert.** You won't miss belt-busting peach cobbler if you have other good-for-you options on hand. Try making grilled fruit kebabs to save 166 calories and score some filling fiber: Slice one peach and one small banana into quarters, thread four pieces fruit each onto two skewers, and brush with one tablespoon honey each. Throw it on the barbecue and grill each side for about four minutes, or until flesh is tender but still firm, and sprinkle with cinnamon.

7 **Build a better burger.** Forget plain ol' white buns and ketchup; the veggies and herbs in these recipes, by J. Kenji López-Alt, Food Lab blogger at SeriousEats.com, deliver good-for-you nutrients—and your cookout guests get a work of art. Tip: Lightly pat burgers into shape, rather than kneading them, for juicier patties.

◆ **Patty-melt burger**

Grill a thin burger patty, and place it on one rye-bread slice—eating open-faced saves yourself some carbs and calories so you can top it with a slice of Swiss cheese and sauerkraut. Put sandwich on a cool part of the grill until the bread is golden brown and cheese is melted. Serve with 2 tablespoons spicy mustard for dipping.

◆ **Pickled-anything burger**

Mix equal parts sugar, white vinegar, and water; bring to boil. Pour over a bowl of sliced veggies. Grill a poblano pepper; cut into strips. While patty grills, top with a slice of low-fat pepper jack cheese. Finish with pickled veg, pepper strips, and fresh cilantro.

◆ **Gyro-esque burger**

For the sauce, stir ½ cup nonfat Greek yogurt with a tablespoon each of lemon juice and fresh chopped mint; season with salt. Grill your patty, and then tuck it into a whole-wheat pita pocket. Finish with a sprinkling of feta cheese, cucumber slices, and some sauce.

BIKINI DIET MEAL PLAN WEEK 9

Turn back to the Month 3 Bikini Diet Meal Plan Cheat Sheet on page 114 for a quick overview on what to eat this week, or go to Chapter 14 page 177 for details on portion sizes and recipes. Remember, you can save a day or two of your Flex Calories and spend them on a few cocktails at happy hour. And if the idea of skipping the bread basket at your fave Italian restaurant depresses you, plan on dining out on your earned day, and allow yourself a little splurge (see page 34 for a reminder about how to plan your earned day).

HOT & HEALTHY WORKOUT WEEK 9

Here's what to do this week:

◆ Morning Cardio Blast Workout 4 to 5 times per week, as soon as you wake up (See page 219.)

◆ Tracy Anderson's Upper Body Blast, twice a week—but not on consecutive days! (See page 220.)

◆ Barry's Bootcamp Total-Body Strength Circuit, twice a week—but not on consecutive days! (See page 219.)

◆ Feel-Good Fitness Day once this week (See page 221.)

◆ Rest and recover—2 days per week, but not on consecutive days!

It's time to achieve A-list tone with Tracy Anderson's Upper-Body Blast routine targeting your arms, shoulders, back, and core. Must-have tool: your lightest weights, because they make it easy to hit tricky angles.

Then for your twice-a-week strength-training circuits, you'll use heavier weights. "This month we get serious. It's time to move into the heavy weights because your strength has increased and you're ready to sculpt that body!" says Barry Jay of Barry's Bootcamp. "The heavy set of weights should be about twice the size of your light set of weights, or about 10 to 12 pounds. You can always drop down to lighter weights if it becomes too much."

(UN)GUILTY PLEASURE: PLAN A GIRLS' NIGHT IN

Socializing may fall to the bottom of your to-do list when you're trying to avoid the calorie temptation you're so often confronted with at happy hours and barbecues, but a Gallup poll finds that the more time you spend mingling, the more happy and less stressed you'll feel. In fact, your mood improves with each hour you spend a day socializing.

To make girl time a priority despite your jam-packed schedule, make a date with your besties to have a weekly viewing party for your latest TV show obsession (our current fave is *Girls*). Hosting the party or bringing your own appetizers to a pal's house to share guarantees that you'll have healthy choices on hand while you're catching up.

DRY-MOUTH ERASER

Alcohol is dehydrating, which is why your mouth becomes parched—and your breath seriously rank—after a boozy night. Get saliva flowing again by adding a few cucumber slices to a glass of water and sipping in the morning after a night out. Cucumbers have a naturally high water content, so it's like getting a double dose of H_2O in one shot.

Here are a couple of recipes for inspiration:

SHRIMP AND BERRY CEVICHE

(SERVES 4)

INGREDIENTS

5 tablespoons (from 2 limes) lime juice
½ cup finely chopped fresh mint leaves
½ cup extra-virgin olive oil
1 teaspoon red wine vinegar
½ teaspoon ground coriander
½ teaspoon crushed red pepper
⅛ teaspoon sugar
1 ¼ pounds (16-20) cooked, shelled, deveined large shrimp, coarsely chopped
1 avocado, chopped
½ seedless (English) cucumber, chopped
4 ounces strawberries, hulled and chopped (about 1 cup)
1 container (6-ounces) blueberries
¼ cup finely chopped red onion
Baked tortilla chips, for serving

DIRECTIONS

◆ In large bowl, whisk together lime juice, mint, oil, vinegar, coriander, red pepper, sugar, and ¼ teaspoon salt.
◆ Add shrimp, avocado, cucumber, strawberries, blueberries, and red onion; fold until well combined.
◆ Cover and refrigerate. Can be made up to 2 hours ahead. Serve with baked tortialla chips.

LAYERED WHITE BEAN AND TOMATO DIP

(SERVES 12)

INGREDIENTS

1 can (28-ounces) whole tomatoes, peeled and drained
2 tablespoons olive oil, divided
1 shallot, finely chopped
1 clove garlic, finely chopped
2 teaspoons sugar

2 sprigs fresh thyme
Salt
Pepper
2 cans (14-ounces each) cannellini beans, rinsed and drained
4 ounces feta cheese, crumbled
⅓ cups light mayonnaise
2 tablespoons lemon juice
1 cup parsley leaves, finely chopped
3 scallions, dark green parts only, thinly sliced
2 tablespoons capers, drained
Crudités, for serving

DIRECTIONS

◆ In bowl, with hands, crush tomatoes into small bits; drain. Discard liquid.
◆ In 2-quart saucepan, heat 1 tablespoon oil on medium. Add shallot and garlic; cook 2 minutes or until golden, stirring. Add tomatoes, sugar, thyme, ⅛ teaspoon salt, and pinch of black pepper. Cook 6 to 8 minutes or until almost dry, stirring. Remove from heat; discard thyme. Cool.
◆ In food processor, pulse beans, feta, mayonnaise, lemon juice, remaining tablespoon oil, and ⅛ teaspoon salt until smooth.
◆ In medium bowl, combine parsley, scallions, and capers.
◆ In 4-cup serving bowl, layer half of bean dip, all of tomato sauce, and half of herb mixture. Top with remaining dip and herb mixture. Cover; refrigerate at least 2 hours or up to 1 day. Serve with crudités.

SUCCESS TRACKER:

Bikini Body Checklist Week 9

❐ I've been using the Bikini Diet strategies when dining out—like custom ordering my salads to help slim them down.

❐ I've been making more Bikini Diet–friendly drink choices at happy hours.

❐ I've been filling up on foods that will fuel me before hitting parties and barbecues so I'm not starving when I arrive.

❐ I've followed the Bikini Diet meal plan.

❐ I've followed the Hot & Healthy Workout plan.

❐ I've made socializing a priority by organizing a TV show viewing party or other weekly get together with the girls.

Week 9 Measurements

Weight _____

Waist _____

Chest _____

Hips _____

This week I feel _____

_____

_____

_____

_____

_____

_____

_____

_____

_____

_____

CHAPTER TEN

MELT YOUR MIDDLE

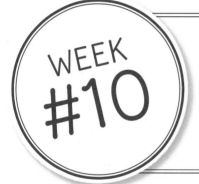

WEEK
#10

THE LOWDOWN You already know the math: You have to cut 3,500 calories to drop one pound. To lose a healthy pound a week, that's 500 calories a day! Which means you need to eat fewer calories than your body burns or up your exercise to burn more calories.

The good news: there are some simple tricks you can do to stoke the fires of your metabolism so your body uses more fuel overall.

Did you know that your body torches calories even when you're not doing anything at all? The fancy term for how much energy your body uses at rest is called your basal metabolism. The thing is, you can actually slow your metabolism and make your body store fat if you eat fewer calories than it needs at rest. Why? Your body feels under attack and fights back to protect its energy by slowing down metabolism and going into starvation mode. That means you'll need to eat even *less* food to maintain your current weight (not to mention to drop pounds). This translates into hunger-induced moodiness as well as the dreaded love handles where your body stores fat. Not exactly the bikini look you were going for when you decided to skimp on food!

The bikini body truth is that getting your sexiest figure doesn't have to feel like torture. This week's Bikini Diet secret is all about how to make your metabolism work in your favor.

This chapter includes:
◆ What to add to your diet rather than what to cut so you can eat well and still lose weight
◆ How switching up your fitness routine helps you fight belly fat
◆ Why *when* you eat may matter just as much as *what* you eat
◆ Three slimming workouts in one from Tracy Anderson

All of these tricks will help your metabolism pick up the pace to melt away stubborn belly fat so you can feel more confident rocking your bikini.

THE TOP 10 TRICKS TO MELT YOUR MIDDLE

1 **Indulge in These Belly-Fat Melting Foods.** Depriving yourself in order to drop pounds sucks, not to mention that it never works. What does: Downing these satisfying superfoods that give your metabolism a kick so you actually burn fat while you eat. Stock your kitchen with these nine belly-fat fighters.
◆ **Avocado** It's high in craving-quelling "good" fat and rich in L-carnitine, an amino acid that fires up your body's engine.
◆ **Cheese** The enzyme known as conjugated linoleic acid in dairy helps your body burn fat. Go with a tangy, creamy kind that satisfies your palate.
◆ **Eggs** Vitamin B12 in the yolk helps your body torch fat.
◆ **Green Tea** It's teeming with catechins, antioxidants that studies show destroy body fat. Plus, caffeine gives your system a metabolic jump.
◆ **Peanut Butter** Creamy or chunky, it's a source of magnesium, which powers cells to metabolize energy efficiently.
◆ **Pickles** A medium pickle is only 7 calories—you'll burn more energy digesting this salty, crunchy veggie.
◆ **Quinoa** Because your body works hard digesting this protein-packed, high in fiber whole grain, you burn off extra calories.
◆ **Sirloin Burger** Made with 90 percent lean beef, it's high in protein, which takes more energy to digest than fat or carbs.
◆ **Yogurt** Regular and low-fat kinds have probiotics, bacteria that may reduce the amount of fat your body absorbs. (See below on how they work to boost your metabolism).

2 **Get A Daily Dose of Probiotics.** Probiotics are the healthy bacteria that live in your gut and aid in weight loss by helping your body digest food and regulate metabolism. If you don't have enough of the "good" bacteria compared to tummy-trouble causing "bad" bacteria in your digestive tract, you might have a tougher time shedding weight. One study found that overweight girls had an imbalance of "good" bacteria in their guts compared to those in the normal-weight range. Experts think an unhealthy balance of gut bacteria may be one culprit for packing on the pounds, according to a study in *BMC Microbiology*.

So how does the ratio of healthy bacteria to the unhealthy kind in your gut get out of whack? Taking antibiotics could kill off both types of bacteria, and poor diet is also one of the most common ways to upset the delicate balance. The key is to eat plenty of fruits and vegetables because they contain *pre*biotics, which the healthy bacteria (aka *pro*biotics) feed on so they can survive and thrive. Prebiotics are those soluable fibers found in veggies such as leeks, garlic, artichokes, oats, and soybeans. Also scan the nutrition label on packaged foods for the ingredient inulin, another form of prebiotics.

The best sources of the healthy bacteria (aka probiotics) are dairy foods such as yogurt (be sure to check the container before buying so it isn't past the expiration date or the bacteria are likely to be dead), cottage cheese, and kefir. If you're lactose intolerant, you can still find probiotics in fermented foods like sauerkraut, barreled pickles (preservatives in the bottled kind kill healthy bacteria), and miso.

You may see probiotics on the labels of unfermented foods, such as coffee and pizza. Avoid marketing hype by buying only products that say *live and active culture* on the label. Steer clear of probiotic items that need to be heated, since cooking those foods could kill the good bacteria.

You could also try taking a probiotics supplement. For overall wellness, look for brands that contain the bacteria strains *Lactobacillus* (acidophilius is the most common type of this strain) and *Bifidobacterium*. Also be sure your supplement supplies at least 1 billion colony-forming units (CFUs) in a day's serving.

3 **Don't Skip—or Skip Out—on Lunch.** This may take some getting used to if you're so busy that you sometimes forget to have lunch, but try making lunch a substantial meal because you'll burn that energy throughout the rest of the day. And eating lunch on the earlier side can help with weight loss. Dieters who ate lunch before 3 p.m. lost 5 pounds more during 20 weeks than those who ate lunch after 3 p.m.—even though both groups were eating about the same amount of calories a day, according to a study in the *International Journal of Obesity*.

Another tip: While you may need to eat out for some client lunches, brown-bagging it may help you achieve your bikini bod more quickly: A study discovered that women who avoid eating out for lunch tended to eat fewer overall calories, according to the *Journal of the Academy of Nutrition and Dietetics*. Study participants who ate lunch out at least weekly also lost five pounds *less* than those who ate lunches brought from home. Dining in restaurants usually means you have less control over ingredients and cooking methods, as well as larger portion sizes—and you learned some tricks on how to eat smarter when eating out in the last chapter. Still, it's a slimming idea to try packing salad with chicken for protein and sliced avocado or sunflower seeds for healthy fats in to-go containers for an easy, portion-controlled midday meal when you can.

4 **Eat Light at Night.** *When* you eat may be just as important for getting your best bikini body as *what* you eat. It turns out that eating late at night really can make you gain weight, according to a study from the University of Pennsylvania. "Your body is actually on a natural rhythm that's ideal to follow in order to help you maintain weight loss," says health coach Ali Shapiro. "Most people rush around, eating breakfast on the go, skipping lunch, and then eating a big dinner."

This week, aim to make your dinner light but high in protein and quality carbs. Now that you're eating breakfast, lunch, and two snacks, you won't be running on empty and feel like you want to binge after work. Bonus: Eating light at night should also allow you to sleep better so you wake up well rested, helping you make smarter food choices and less likely to reach for a sugary pick-me-up out of exhaustion.

5 **Ditch Extreme Dieting or Fasts.** Following the Cosmo Bikini Diet puts you on track to shed pounds and keep them off for good. Don't be tempted to fast in order to make the number on the scale drop faster, because it could backfire by sending your body into starvation mode and slowing your metabolism. Sure, you'll lose lots of water weight by fasting or doing a liquid-only diet, but you'll also lose muscle because you're depriving your body of essential nutrients such as protein. That only sets you up to pack on more body fat later because you'll have less muscle overall, which naturally burns extra calories and boosts metabolism.

"The main driver of metabolism is the amount of muscle you have, so eating too few calories makes you lose muscle and ultimately lowers your metabolism," says Terry Shaw, MA, a licensed dietician and nutritionist for the Lake Austin Spa in Austin, Texas. "A pound of muscle burns an average of 30 calories a day just to stay alive, while a pound of fat burns only one calorie. So simply gaining one pound of muscle means you'll use an extra 30 calories a day effortlessly, to help your body shed three pounds of fat in a year."

6 **Focus on Losing Inches Rather Than Losing Pounds.** To really rev your metabolism and make long-lasting changes to your body's shape, make building muscle and losing fat your MO rather than obsessing about losing pounds. "When it comes to slimming down, the tape measure may be a better friend than the scale," says Shaw. "Even though muscle weighs more than fat, it's much more compact—a pound of muscle takes up one-third of the space that a pound of fat takes up." This is why a

130-pound woman with 18 percent body fat is apt to fit into a size 2, while a woman who weighs the exact same weight of 130 but that has 26 percent body fat may wear a size 12.

And whether you're an apple or a pear shape matters when it comes to your health: If most of your weight is around your waist rather than your hips, your odds of getting Type 2 diabetes and heart disease rises. That's because your middle is where visceral adipose tissue is stored, and this type of deep belly fat may contribute to insulin resistance and mess with carbohydrate metabolism. You should be noticing that your waist has shrunk after measuring and recording it every week. (And hopefully you've been recording your hip measurements too.)

To find out if you're carrying extra belly fat, divide your waist measurement by your hip measurement in inches to measure your waist-to-hip ratio. You're carrying extra belly fat if your ratio is .08 or greater, so be extra focused on building muscle to help you burn fat faster and boost your metabolism.

7 **Crank Up Your Cardio.** If you want to lose your spare tire, adding intervals to your cardio routine is key. That's why it's important to switch up your intensity for your morning cardio session rather than sticking to the same steady pace. Whether you're walking, jogging, biking, or swimming, boost the intensity (and calorie burn!) by alternating between a fast pace for one minute and a slower recovery pace for one minute. Keep it going for about 15 to 20 minutes, and follow with a cool down and light stretching.

8 **Add Some Resistance.** To melt fat faster, make sure you're doing your two weight lifting and two toning sessions a week in addition to the a.m. cardio intervals. You'll build muscle while burning fat, and now you know that muscle boosts your metabolism because it torches calories all day long.

"The worst thing you can do is cut back on your calories and not do strength training because you'll lose muscle tone," says Shaw. Bonus: Research finds that strength training also builds the type of muscle that helps regulate blood sugar to tame your appetite.

9 **Sip Some Iced Water.** Sipping water is an appetite-taming move because it's easy to mistake being thirsty for being hungry. Drinking it cold may also help speed your metabolism, according to a study in *The Journal of Clinical Endocrinology and Metabolism*. In fact, drinking about 6 cups of icy H_2O daily could boost your resting metabolism by about 50 calories a day, which means you could shed up to five extra pounds in a year. One theory is that sipping the cold stuff makes your body work harder to warm it up and therefore burns more calories.

10 **Make your Diet Pump Some Iron.** Women need more iron in their diets than guys do in part because you lose iron every month during your period. Being low on iron can make you feel tired and your metabolism sluggish. After all, the mineral is needed to deliver oxygen to your cells for energy and to burn fat. You can boost levels in your body by eating iron-rich foods such as grass-fed red meats, liver, fortified cereals (like Total), and oysters, as well as taking iron supplements.

Also practice smart food pairing by combining non-animal sources of iron-rich foods with vitamin C–packed produce to help boost iron absorption. Examples of iron-rich plant foods are black beans and spinach, and vitamin C–rich foods include broccoli, red bell peppers, tomatoes and lemons. Iron helps transport oxygen throughout your body to keep you from feeling sluggish and also strengthens your immune system. Food Fix: The RDA is 18 mg of iron for women. Simply adding a side of cooked spinach or lentils to a meal offers 6 mg—sprinkle it with lemon juice or mix with chopped tomatoes to boost the mineral's absorption.

BIKINI DIET MEAL PLAN WEEK 10

Turn back to the Month 3 Bikini Diet Meal Plan Cheat Sheet on page 114 for a quick overview on what to eat this week, or go to Chapter 14 page 177 for details on portion sizes and Bikini Diet recipes. Find ways to fit into this month's meal plan some of the metabolism-boosting foods listed in this chapter (see page 131) to help melt more fat from your middle. Like if you always have a cup of coffee with breakfast, go for green tea instead this week. Or make your burger lettuce wrap with ground sirloin and serve with a few pickle spears.

HOT & HEALTHY WORKOUT WEEK 10

Here's what to do this week:

◆ Morning Cardio Blast Workout 4 to 5 times per week, as soon as you wake up (See page 222.)
◆ Tracy Anderson's Three Slimming Workouts in One routine, twice a week—but not on consecutive days! (See page 223.)
◆ Barry's Bootcamp Total-Body Strength Circuit, twice a week—but not on consecutive days! (See page 223.)
◆ Feel-Good Fitness Day once this week (See page 224.)
◆ Rest and recover—2 days per week, but not on consecutive days!

This week's Tracy Anderson's Three Slimming Workouts in One routine targets a trio of body parts, so you can get trim and sculpted in a third of the time. All these exercises use a hand towel, which Tracy and her celeb clients swear by. Gripping it engages your muscles even more, so you tone up more quickly.

You're now in the home stretch, so put together a new playlist to keep you pumped during your sweat sessions. "Creating a playlist of your favorite songs makes working out feel more fun and can really push you to exercise harder and for longer," says Barry Jay, who puts the spotlight on music in his cardio-and-weights combo classes to create a night club party atmosphere that his students rave about.

(UN)GUILTY PLEASURE: USE YOUR VACATION DAYS

One reason French women don't get fat? They take their vacation days and savor them. Americans get a measly 14 vacation days a year and take only 12, compared to our French or Spanish counterparts who use all of the 30 vacation days given to them, according to Expedia's Vacation Deprivation survey.

If you're thinking about skipping your summer vacation in order to look good at work, know that you're not doing your boss any favors. In fact, leaving vacation days unused can hurt your health and lower productivity. Here are some ways that skimping on vacation is bad for your mind *and* your body:

- ◆ **You're more apt to feel blue.** Women who don't take regular vacations are up to three times more likely to be depressed compared with their counterparts who take more time off, discovered researchers from the Marshfield Clinic, in Wisconsin.
- ◆ **You'll hurt your ticker.** Women who go on vacation have a 50 percent lower risk of heart attack, according to the Framingham Heart Study.
- ◆ **You'll boost stress levels.** You need to carve out time off to keep a healthy balance: Stress squashes your immune system and has been shown to increase your odds of suffering from adrenal dysfunction, headaches and irritable bowel syndrome—not to mention makes you fat!
- ◆ **You'll age faster.** Working too much without taking vacation to help your body recharge can elevate levels of chronic stress so much that it can actually speed up the aging process. Research in the journal *Biological Psychiatry* shows that people who are severely stressed have shorter telomeres — the outermost part of the chromosome that gets shorter as we grow older. You're too young to look old!

So whether you're craving a staycation where you learn a new skill (cooking classes?); a girlfriend getaway that includes plenty of spas, shopping, and female bonding; a romantic vacation where you rent a house on the beach with your honey; or a solo trip where you take time to reflect or explore a far-flung place, just be sure you don't let your days off go to waste by spending them in front of your computer like you probably do almost every other day. This week, do something nice for yourself and your slimmer bikini body by taking time out to plan your summer vacation and giving your boss advance notice. You're much more likely to pack your bags once you've made your vacation public and put the dates in the calendar.

SUCCESS TRACKER:

Bikini Body Checklist Week 10

☐ I've stocked my kitchen with belly-fat-melting foods.

☐ I've added more probiotics and iron to my diet.

☐ I've sipped at least 6 cups of ice water daily.

☐ I've been smarter about my meal timing and making sure I don't eat dinner too late at night.

☐ I've followed the Bikini Diet meal plan.

☐ I've followed the Hot & Healthy Workout plan.

☐ I've planned a vacation and told my boss when I'm taking time off so the dates are in the calendar.

Week 10 Measurements

Weight_____

Waist_____

Chest_____

Hips_____

This week I feel _____

_____

_____

_____

_____

_____

_____

_____

_____

_____

_____

CHAPTER ELEVEN

SLASH SNEAKY SOURCES OF SUGAR

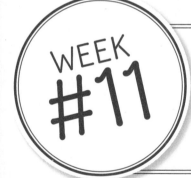

WEEK #11

THE LOWDOWN This week you'll learn how to cut back on added sugars like high fructose corn syrups that have been put in during processing as opposed to natural sugars that are found normally in food, like fructose in fruit.

If you lower your added sugar intake by just two little teaspoons per day (and you'll hardly miss them!), you'll keep yourself from consuming a five-pound bag of sugar over the course of the year. Hold a five-pound bag of sugar and try envisioning all that sweet stuff that would have been going into your body. That's the equivalent of guzzling more than 90 cans of soda. (Drinking just one soda a day is like ingesting more than 35 pounds of sugar a year and equals an extra 15 pounds or more of weight gain.) We'll show you how to lighten up without having to sacrifice dessert!

You'll also find out whether or not added sugars *really* make you crave more sweets; the real deal on the juicing trend; and how to make your postworkout high last.

HOW TO SPOT HIDDEN SOURCES OF SUGAR

It's not that we don't love the sweet stuff just as much as the next girl (sometimes we just gotta give in to the calling for a melt-in-your-mouth glazed doughnut or a chewy Twizzler fix), but the problem is that many of us unknowingly overdose on sugar.

"The average American diet packs more than 140 pounds of added sugars a year that's been dumped into processed foods and drinks," says Jacob Teitelbaum, MD, author of *Beat Sugar Addiction Now!* "Eating sugar causes blood sugar to surge, insulin to spike, and fat to get deposited throughout your body." Sugar is kind of like crack: It gives you a quick high when blood sugar rises, followed by the buzzkill that happens when it drops shortly afterward. The more of the sweet stuff you eat, the more you crave it and the more you get trapped in this ongoing cycle.

The sneaky thing about sugar is that it lurks everywhere in our diet, and it's not always easy to spot. It wouldn't be rocket science to try to cut out food with added sugars if they were all called "sugar" on nutrition labels. But sugars by many different names are added to all kinds of packaged foods during processing, including many items that you might not even realize contain sugar (think: breads, pasta sauces, salad dressings, slaws, and soups, etc.)

While eating foods that naturally contain sugar, such as fruits, is healthy, downing too many foods with added sugars (like muffins, sodas, and ice cream) leads to empty calories and weight gain. In addition, man-made sweeteners, such as the high-fructose corn syrup (HFCS) added to many processed foods, have been linked to high blood pressure. To figure out if a food item has *added* sugars, you have to scour the ingredient list. Here is a list of added sugar by some other names:

Agave nectar*	Corn syrup solids	Maltodextrin
Barley malt	Dextrose	Maltose
Cane-juice crystals	Fruit juice concentrate	Molasses
Cane sugar	Glucose	Organic brown rice syrup
Caramel	HFCS	Sorghum syrup
Carob syrup	Malt syrup	Sucrose

*Often touted as "all natural," the kind added to packaged foods tends to have even more fructose than high-fructose corn syrup!

So if you see any of these added sugar ingredients on a nutrition label—especially if it appears at or near the top of the list—you might want to leave it on the shelf in favor of a product that does not contain added sugar, or that doesn't list an added sugar as one of its main ingredients.

Just because you're not eating candy bars doesn't mean your diet isn't high in added sugar—a definite bikini-bod wrecker. Some common foods that seem healthy—such as yogurt, kefir, smoothies, salad dressings, and whole-grain cereals—can be loaded with added sugar. Case in point: It's typical for a sweetened (even whole-grain) cereal to have 12 to 17 grams of sugar or more per serving. That's like piling on three to four teaspoons worth of sugar. The recommended daily allowance (RDA) for a 1600-calorie diet is only about 24 grams, or six teaspoons, of *added* sugar per day. (To figure out how many teaspoons you're eating, just divide the grams of sugar on the food label by four.) Whole grains, like whole wheat by itself, have no sugar, but often some healthy-looking cereals such as granola have between 15 and 20 grams of added sugar per serving.

This week try playing detective and reading the ingredient list to see if you find *added* sugars in the foods that you eat often. Then, swap in lower-sugar substitutes. If your flavored yogurt has added sugars listed (think: evaporated cane juice rather than the naturally sweet lactose from dairy), go for the plain, unsweetened kind instead. Besides cutting down on processed foods and eating more whole foods, such as fruits and nuts, here are some easy ways to slash sneaky sources of sugar:

◆ **Bread** You may not think of bread as being sugar-heavy, but many brands of both white and whole wheat have surprisingly high levels of HFCS. Go for breads that list whole grains up top on the nutrition label (remember, unbleached wheat flour does not count as a whole grain, but sprouted wheat, barley, millet, sprouts, etc. do. See page 88 in Chapter 6 for more about decoding bread food labels).

◆ **Cereal** Switch from a sugar-sweetened cereal such as Honey Nut Cheerios (12 g) to a non-sweetened version such as regular Cheerios (1 g).

◆ **Juices** Cut back on sugar in fruit juice by pouring only half a glass and adding water to fill. Or instead of gulping processed and watered-down orange juice, eat a whole orange instead. You'll get to enjoy the fiber and other nutrients of the fresh fruit and the flavor of the juice.

◆ **Yogurt** Opt for plain yogurt over the flavored kind, and then toss in fruit for natural sweetness to get more nutritional bang for your buck.

◆ **Soft Drinks** A big source of added fructose. Try swapping soda for seltzer mixed with berries or frozen lemon wedges. Fruit has less fructose than processed food while being packed with vitamins and minerals to help lessen sugar's harmful effects.

◆ **Pastries** Another big source of added fructose. Swap muffins for oatmeal topped with banana slices.

◆ **Bottled Sauces and Dressings** Use a dry rub instead of sugar-heavy sauce to add flavor when grilling or marinating meat. (Both barbecue sauce and Italian dressing, for example, could have 21 grams of sugar per 8 ounces—and the low-fat kind could have twice as much.) You can make your own sugar-free rub by mixing together 1 tableshoon black pepper; 2 teaspoon chili powder; and ½ teaspoon each salt, cayenne and granulated garlic.

◆ **Pasta sauces** A cup of marinara sauce has about 15 grams of sugar—more than half your daily limit! To cut back on sugar, try using half as much sauce on your pasta and adding chunks of fresh tomato.

5 WAYS SUGAR CAN BE TOXIC

Here's more motivation to cut back on sugar.

1 **Sugar makes you fat.** Sugar in the form of HFCS is found in many processed snacks, and Americans have upped their consumption of it by more than 250 percent in the last 15 years, says Dr. Teitelbaum. HFCS has been blamed for Americans' widening waistlines, and a recent study uncovers that it may trigger overeating. When scientists at the Yale School of Medicine did brain scans on healthy, non-obese people after eating a treat made with HFCS, they discovered that the sweet stuff failed to make subjects feel satisfied or full, possibly prompting them to down more calories later on.

2 **Sugar is a diabetes culprit.** Diabetes rates are surging, and the main offender behind the disease may actually be sugar rather than obesity, finds a recent study. When researchers scoured the data from more than 175 countries, they found that for every additional 150 calories of sugar a person had access to a day (about as much as in a 12-ounce can of soda), diabetes rates went up 1 percent—even after controlling for obesity and physical activity. The study basically shows that diabetes may have less to do with the number on the scale and more to do with the amount of sugar you consume.

3 **Sugar ups your odds of cancer.** High blood sugar levels have been linked to an increase in a prime cancer culprit—a protein called beta-catenin, according to the journal *Molecular Cell*.

4 **Sugar could hurt your heart.** Having a sweet tooth may increase your blood pressure as well as your belly fat. In a study of 4,528 adults, people who consumed more than 74 grams of added fructose a day (about the amount in 2.5 sweetened soft drinks) were 87 percent more likely to have severely elevated blood pressure than those getting less, according to researchers at the University of Denver. Fructose can reduce cell's nitrous oxide production so blood vessels have to work harder to relax and dilate, or it may stimulate the nervous system, both of which could increase blood pressure.

5 **Sugar can cause wrinkles.** A study found that people with higher sugar in their bloodstreams had more lines and wrinkles than their less sugared-up counterparts. Researchers believe that sugar attacks collagen, the stuff that helps keep skin firm and smooth.

CAN EATING FAKE SUGARS MAKE YOU CRAVE MORE SWEETS?

Processed foods packed with sugar substitutes such as aspartame or saccharin may prompt you to eat more calories later on. Why? Artificial sweeteners taste even more sweet than the sugar you get from nature (think: fruits), so it's like giving fuel to your sweet tooth to keep those cravings coming. Plus, they could make you hungrier because your body expects calories when it tastes something sweet and sends "feed me" signals to your brain when you're not getting any substantial or filling calories from sugar-free candies, beverages, and other snacks. That may make you want to keep noshing until your body gets those expected calories.

Moreover, sweet substitutes such as sugar alcohols (like maltitol found in sugar-free chocolates) can cause gas and bloating. Aspartame (aka NutraSweet) has been linked with headaches, memory loss, and even heart palpitations.

THE REAL DEAL ON THE JUICING TREND

Since we're talking about how even healthy foods can be packed with sugar, we should mention the juicing trend, since even **a small glass of orange juice has as much sugar as a can of soda**—no joke. We're not saying that juicing is on par with junk food, it's just that it's better to juice responsibly if you want to cut out sneaky sources of sugar. While juicing veggies is an excellent way to pack even higher levels of healthy antioxidants into your diet than you would be able to get by eating them as solid foods (you'd have to eat *sooo* much more of the solid kind!), juicing high volumes of fruit already naturally loaded with fructose (even though it's natural!) can easily send you on a sugar high. Juicing an orange isn't bad (you'll get a healthy dose of nutrients like vitamin C along with that natural sugar), but juicing a few oranges along with fructose-packed mangoes or bananas in high volumes that you normally wouldn't consume as whole fruits can really up your sugar intake even though you think you're being healthy.

You may have seen pics of celebs such as Blake Lively and Nicole Richie sipping on green juice, and that may be because drinking your veggies is gaining in popularity, with organic-juice bar chains opening in more locations, and sales of pricey juicers such as Vitamix surging by more than 52 percent last year. The juicing trend can

If you really don't like your coffee black or are looking for a sugar-free baking blend, stevia is an alternative. The calorie-free sweetener comes from the leaves of the South American stevia plant. Some brands of stevia have a bitter aftertaste if not filtered properly, so you might try switching brands if you don't like your first taste. One to try: NuStevia from NuNaturals is sweet, not bitter, and comes in single-serving packets; bottles of tablets that are easy to toss in your purse; liquid droppers that fully dissolve in cold drinks like iced tea, and baking blends so you can try swapping for sugar in recipes. (*$9.99 for 100 packets of NuStevia; nunaturals.com*)

BIKINI DIET MEAL PLAN WEEK 11

Turn back to the Month 3 Bikini Diet Meal Plan Cheat Sheet on page 114 for a quick overview on what to eat this week, or go to Chapter 14 page 177 for details on portion sizes and recipes. Remember to do your detective work this week and read food labels to uncover whether sugar by any other name appears at the top of the ingredi-

make it easier to fit whole foods into your diet so you're less apt to rely on processed foods. It's also a quick way to get the recommended five daily servings of produce in a single glass.

Remember, **mashing up some veggies with your fruits can cut back on sugar while giving you a high dose of nutrients,** since juices made from sweet fruits only can put you on sugar overload if you drink too much (more than a glass a day). If you find vegetables hard to swallow, your spinach

or kale might go down more easily in a juice blended with, say, apples or pineapples for added sweetness. You might try this recipe for a **Beet Juice Endurance Enhancer** from chef Andres Meraz of The Ritz-Carlton South Beach, who recently lost 40 pounds in part from kicking off a healthier diet by juicing:

1 red beet
1 chopped carrot
1 chopped red apple
½ cup cold water

This juice packs a lot of nutrients because carrots

have beta-carotene for eye health and apples provide easily-digestible carbs and natural sugar for energy. Some research finds that beet juice may help power your muscles so you can workout longer and harder.

It's best to add a glass of juice to a meal rather than to use it as a liquid meal replacement because, while juices are packed with immune-boosting antioxidants, they're lacking in the healthy fats and protein that make for balanced snacks and meals.

ent list. Swap out any foods you find are high in added sugars for lower sugar alternatives, like plain yogurt for the flavored kind. While the average American downs 88 grams of added sugars a day, the Cosmo Bikini Diet has your back by giving you healthy meal plans well within the 24 grams of added sugar daily limit (no more than 6 teaspoons)—the rest of the sugar grams all come from natural sources, like fructose in fresh fruits or lactose in milk.

HOT & HEALTHY WORKOUT WEEK 11

Here's what to do this week:
◆ Morning Cardio Blast Workout 4 to 5 times per week, as soon as you wake up. (See page 225.)
◆ Tracy Anderson's Your Butt, Only Better routine, twice a week—but not on consecutive days! (See page 226.)
◆ Barry's Bootcamp Total-Body Strength Circuit, twice a week—but not on consecutive days! (See page 225.)
◆ Feel-Good Fitness Day once this week (See page 227.)
◆ Rest and recover—2 days per week, but not on consecutive days!

You'll be ready to slip into those tiny bikini bottoms, thanks to the four moves from Tracy Anderson's Your Butt, Only Better routine. Targeting your glutes won't be nearly as tricky as craning to admire your cute rear view will be.

Think you can increase your weights to 12 pounds this week for Barry's Bootcamp Total-Body Strength Circuit? Then go for it! Rather than bulking up, you'll be sculpting even more lean muscle to keep igniting your metabolism.

(UN)GUILTY PLEASURE: MAKE YOUR POST EXERCISE HIGH LAST

There are plenty of science-proven tricks for making your workout feel pleasurable rather than painful. Try these four ways to put the fun back into shaping up, and to prolong exercise's feel-good effects.

1 **Take a whiff.** Engage your sense of smell to reap an extra mood boost during your workout. Women who inhaled extracts taken from the armpits of anonymous male volunteers felt more relaxed, according to a study in *Biological Reproduction*. Don't have a sweaty man to work out with? Hop on a treadmill next to a sweaty guy. You could banish calories *and* tension.

2 **Maximize your postworkout high.** Exercise can boost mood-elevating neurotransmitters and endorphins to give you a buzz for up to an hour after your sweat session is over. To make it last longer, steer clear of doing things that will stress you out, such as battling a company about a credit card bill dispute, and tackle things that you

know you can finish, such as writing an ideas memo for a project that you're excited about. You'll ward off a buzzkill and prolong that feeling of accomplishment. Bonus: Moving your body helps active your right brain, which is the intuitive, creative side, so you're likely to come up with more imaginative solutions to problems.

3 **Ease muscle soreness.** After a killer workout, try an old-fashioned hot soak with Epsom salt. It's packed with magnesium, a mineral that regulates hundreds of enzymes in your body to help ease everything from cramps to headaches to irritability. Pour 1 cup of Epsom salt into hot water for a muscle relaxant that will help relieve cramps and joint pain.

4 **Take a breather.** Another trick for prolonging your exercise buzz and speeding muscle recovery is to do a five-minute yoga breather immediately following your workout. Breathing smoothly and steadily while doing the postures helps lower your heart rate and blood pressure to maximize feelings of relaxation. Studies show that yoga also lowers levels of a neurotransmitter associated with anxiety. Try unwinding with a standing forward bend followed by a seated butterfly (with the soles of your feet together), and finish with a seated spinal twist.

SUCCESS TRACKER:

Bikini Body Checklist Week 11

☐ I've slashed sneaky sources of sugar by scouring food labels for sugar by other names and eating less packaged food and more whole foods.

☐ I'm replacing soda and other liquid sugar bombs with water and more nutritious green juices.

☐ I've followed the Bikini Diet meal plan.

☐ I've followed the Hot & Healthy Workout plan.

☐ I've made my workouts more enjoyable by trying some of the tricks to make my postworkout high last longer.

Week 11 Measurements

Weight _____

Waist _____

Chest _____

Hips _____

This week I feel _____

_____

_____

_____

_____

_____

_____

_____

_____

_____

_____

_____

CHAPTER TWELVE

FOODS THAT FLATTEN YOUR TUMMY

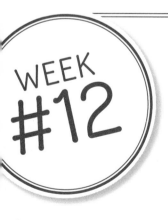

WEEK #12

THE LOWDOWN Congratulations! You're in the very last week of the Cosmo Bikini Diet. You should be feeling much lighter and more energized than when you started just 11 weeks ago. While you've already done most of the hard work and your body is tighter and stronger, there are still some tricks that you can try this week to banish beach-day bloat and make your stomach look its flattest.

You'll learn which foods to eat (and which to skip) to get your sexiest bikini body before hitting the beach. You'll also score a checklist of beach-bag essentials.

You're probably feeling so good now that you wouldn't dream of returning to (or starting!) a lifestyle of guzzling beers and downing greasy fries while sitting on your butt all day. Still, to keep you motivated to continue taking care of yourself for the long haul, we've included a special section on how to create your own Bliss List (see this week's (Un)Guilty Pleasure on page 152). You can reach for it as a quick pick-me-up (in place of food and drinks) for the rest of your life, and it will remind you to do one feel-good thing for yourself a day. You're now in the home stretch!

6 TUMMY-FLATTENING FOODS

Big beach day ahead? These bloat-fighting foods will get you a flatter tummy by the afternoon to keep you feeling foxy and confident.

1. ASPARAGUS This green veggie is rich in calcium and magnesium, two nutrients that help your body digest food properly. It's also a natural diuretic (which means it helps eliminate water retention).

2. COTTAGE CHEESE Spread some (no salt added) onto whole-grain toast for a satisfying lunch option that won't round you out. It's easy to digest, and the fiber push from the grains will help normalize digestion.

3. CUCUMBER WATER Sounds counterintuitive, but dehydration can inflate your stomach since air builds up in your colon, backing up your digestive tract. Drink lots of H_2O with cucumber, a natural diuretic.

4. FISH Fish like salmon, halibut, sardines, and tuna are rich in omega-3 fats—the good fats that speed up digestion, so food exits the stomach faster so you don't feel all bloated and full.

5. GARLIC Add flavor to food with chopped garlic instead of salt. It helps your liver filter toxins, so your body can metabolize fat properly.

6. GRAPEFRUIT The faster you eat, the more air you let into your body, which puffs you out. Luckily, this fruit is challenging to eat, slowing you down. Use a serrated spoon to dig out each delicious bite.

6 BIG, FAT BLOATERS

Stay away from these unless you want to see more of your muffin top.

1. CARBONATED DRINKS Bubbly drinks that contain sugar or carbs can cause a distended belly. The carbon dioxide from the fizz also makes your stomach expand so you look and feel puffy. Nix soda, beer, and champagne on beach day and the night before.

2. CHEWING GUM The bubbalicious stuff makes you gulp in extra air, creating a tummy pooch. Instead of chomping on gum, try a natural de-bloater and breath-freshener in one: Peppermint oil capsules can kill bacteria that causes stinky breath and bloating, and also aid digestion.

3. REFINED CARBS They may increase insulin levels, which causes fat to be stored in your gut. Skip white pasta, rice, and bread. Instead go for quinoa, sweet potatoes, brown rice, and other whole grains.

4. SALT Overdosing on salt is a weight-loss roadblock because it can make you retain water and your stomach swell. To cut back on sodium, steer clear of Chinese food, processed meats, canned soups, ketchup, frozen microwave meals, and soy sauce. Another sneaky source of sodium is found in salad dressing. Banish bloat by making your own dressing (see the Healthy Balsamic Dressing recipe on page 165).

5. SPICY DISHES Adding heat to your food with chili powder or hot sauces can boost the release of stomach acid, triggering inflammation and bloat. Try adding flavor to food with spices that are gentler on your tummy, such as basil and rosemary.

6. SUGAR-FREE SWEETS Sorbitol, an artificial sweetener found in some diet drinks, gums, and hard candies, is difficult for your body to digest and can cause bloating and indigestion. Though it might be tempting to reach for artificially-sweetened cookies or suck on sugar-free candy, have naturally sweet options on hand instead, such as frozen grapes or blueberries.

QUICK AND EASY BELLY-FLATTENING RECIPES

Solve your most challenging beach-day bloat dilemmas by mixing up these tummy-flattening snacks before you hit the surf and sand.

1 **Nosh on a slimming salad.** For a triple dose of natural diuretics that will help you shed extra water weight, toss half of a sliced cucumber with ¼ cup parsley and 1 tablespoon lemon juice.

2 **Go for a hydrating treat.** Remember how dehydration can build up air in your stomach? Avoid getting parched by noshing on fruits—they're natural hydrators since they're at least 60 percent water. Melons, papaya, and mangos are especially good because they also contain potassium, which helps regulate your body's balance of fluids and minerals. Cut a cantaloupe in half, scoop out the seeds, and fill with sliced papaya or mango for a quenching treat.

3 **Sip a digestion-helper smoothie.** Blend together 3 cups each spinach and kale, 2 kiwis, 1 thumb-sized bit of ginger root and ½ cup cold water, suggests chef Andres Meraz of The Ritz-Carlton South Beach in Miami. Green leafy vegetables like spinach are especially high in magnesium, which helps regulate blood sugar to tame appetite. Kiwis have been found to ease symptoms of irritable bowel syndrome such as bloating; while ginger soothes your stomach and eases digestion (for when you need to do some detoxing).

BIKINI DIET MEAL PLAN WEEK 12

Turn back to the Month 3 Bikini Diet Meal Plan Cheat Sheet on page 114 for a quick overview on what to eat this week, or go to Chapter 14 page 177 for details on portion sizes and recipes. Don't forget that you can always swap in any of the snack suggestions in this book in place of any of the snacks or Flex Calorie suggestions outlined in the monthly meal plan—so go ahead and customize however you want. For example, try having the hydrating treat mentioned above (½ cantaloupe with seeds scooped out and filled with sliced papaya or mango) and count it as your Flex calories.

HOT & HEALTHY WORKOUT WEEK 12

Here's what to do this week:

◆ Morning Cardio Blast Workout 4 to 5 times per week, as soon as you wake up (See page 228.)
◆ Tracy Anderson's Whoa! Nice Abs Toning routine, twice a week—but not on consecutive days! (See page 229.)

- Barry's Bootcamp Total-Body Strength Circuit twice a week—but not on consecutive days! (See page 228.)
- Feel-Good Fitness Day once this week (See page 230.)
- Rest and recover—2 days per week, but not on consecutive days!

Say hello to your amazing core, and say "see ya" to crunches with Tracy Anderson's toning tummy moves. Turn up the music and shift with the beat when doing these exercises. Work up to sets that last for one song.

"You can see the finish line, so now really go for it," says Barry Jay of Barry's Bootcamp. "It's the final week of your challenge of doing the Morning Cardio Blasts without stopping and upping the number of push-ups you can do on your toes. Since this *is* the Cosmo Bikini Diet workout, buy yourself a bikini and put it on when you're working out at home to push yourself harder."

TOP 10 BEACH BAG ESSENTIALS

You've made many healthy, feel-good changes to get your best bikini body, and now all you have to do is pack your beach bag and go! Make sure you bring along these must-haves for your next pool party or day on the sand to look and feel your best.

1. SEXY BIKINI You've worked hard on your body. Now show it off by treating yourself to a bikini that makes you feel as fabulous as you look. Ruffles on top can make a small chest look bigger, boy shorts give more bottom coverage, and high-cut bottoms elongate legs.

2. COMFY FLIP-FLOPS Ditch those cheap plastic flip-flops that are likely to break and leave your feet burning up in the sand (or on the pavement). Instead, go for a padded, stylish pair that won't leave your dogs barking.

3. CHEMICAL-FREE SUNSCREEN While religiously slathering on sunscreen is a healthy move, it's best to steer clear of formulas that use *chemical* UV blockers. Research finds that common sunscreen ingredients such as octinoxate and oxybenzone may be endocrine disrupters (translation: they could mess with your hormones). Instead, go for brands that contain natural, *physical* sun blockers, such as titanium dioxide or zinc oxide. Eclipse SPF 50 protects with both zinc and titanium dioxide, come in lightly tinted formulas and is water resistant (innovativeskincare.com).

4. A STYLISH HAT You can get wrinkle-causing DNA damage from UVA rays even on cloudy days, so it's best not to rely on sunscreen alone to protect your skin from harmful rays. Try one that also has built-in sun protection, such as the Frankie Fedora (wallaroohats.com). The hat blocks 97.5% of harmful UV rays, and it's also a super simple fix for bad hair days.

5. **LEAVE-IN HAIR CONDITIONER** Apply at the beach to protect strands from the sun's rays. White Sands The Cure 24/7 Hair Cell Renewal can be used on wet or dry hair and is small enough to throw right in your purse or beach bag (whitesandsproducts.com).

6. **TINTED LIP BALM** The skin on your lips is very sensitive and needs sun protection too! A sweet way to protect your kisser on the beach is to use Fresh's Sugar Tinted Treatment Lip Treatment with SPF. It's made with real sugar (a natural humectant that helps keep lips moisturized) and age-fighting vitamins A, C, and E. Try it in the Coral shade, which is a pretty, sheer dark peach that's perfect for sunny days.

7. **HEALTHY SNACKS** By now you probably wouldn't even think of leaving your house without a few good-for-you snacks like an orange or a small baggie of nuts. For another beach-portable idea, check out the new Chia Squeeze Snack. It is made of organic chia seeds and fruit and vegetable purees, has healthy omega-3s, and comes in an easy-to-squeeze pouch that doesn't need to be refrigerated (mammachia.com).

8. **COOL SHADES** Make sure the shape of your glasses matches the shape of your face to best enhance your features. Like if you have a square-shaped face, go for angular, square-shaped lenses instead of oval or cat-eyed shapes. And your eyeballs can get sunburned too, so look for lenses that have 100 percent UV protection.

9. **BPA-FREE WATER BOTTLE** Hey, you need something to carry your de-bloating cucumber water. Bobble Iced water bottles are dishwasher safe; free of BPA, phthalates and PVC; and fit neatly into most car cup holders (available at Best Buy and Old Navy or waterbobble.com).

10. **FRESHENING WIPES** For those times when you're going straight to happy hour from the beach, it's a good idea to carry some cleansing wipes to swipe away the sweat and sand. Any will do, but Shobha's Rosewater Freshening Cloths for the face, body, and bikini are paraben and artificial-fragrance free and smell like, well, roses. Plus, they come in single packets that you can easily toss into your beach bag (myshobha.com).

(UN)GUILTY PLEASURE: MAKE A BLISS LIST

"We all need a go-to list of immediate action items to help us get calm and centered, especially on those chaotic, overwhelming days," says Kelly Newsome, yoga instructor and founder of Higher Ground Yoga (highergroundyoga.com) based in Washington, D.C. "In fact, practicing daily bliss can calm your internal chaos, creating more space and patience for your relationships and your work, and can help give you the energy and confidence to reach your weight-loss goals."

Newsome suggests writing a Bliss List, an inventory of things that help you feel your best. Focus on what's easy and doable daily, but also include a few splurges too. "Put your Bliss List in a visible place, and do at least one every day this week," says Newsome. "Write about your experience for a few minutes each day to help you discover ways to fit more joy into your life." See Newsome's Bliss List suggestions below, and brainstorm your own personal happiness helpers that you can turn to daily.

1. Make a date with yourself to see a movie, take a painting class, or to do something else you enjoy but never get around to doing. Don't stand yourself up.
2. Sing out loud. Loudly.
3. Have a two-minute dance party.
4. Take a restorative yoga class.
5. Be still for at least 5 to 10 minutes.
6. Power off your computer at night to keep you from getting sucked into the World Wide Web. You'll be amazed at what else you'll find to do with those lost hours, such as finally finishing that book you've been meaning to read!
7. Use markers or colored pencils to draw, doodle, and hone your inner creativity.
8. Sign out of email and social sites for at least one hour, especially while working on another task. The focus will help your brain feel and perform better!
9. At the end of every day, write out three things you are thankful for.
10. Write a dream list. Keep dreaming.
11. Read poetry.
12. Find a happy photo from childhood. Scan it and make it your new screensaver.
13. Rename your "to do" list a "get to do" list.
14. Make a list of people in your "choir," who always support you. Reach out to connect with one of them. If you don't reach them, think of them for 30 seconds.
15. Say no to what you don't say "hell yes" to.
16. Paint something, be it a picture or a piece of furniture, to add a splash of color to your home.
17. Make the damn massage appointment.
18. Use your favorite candle or essential oil.
19. Use a mantra to refocus your energy.
20. Notice when you say to yourself "I should." Stop.
21. Buy beautiful flowers for yourself.
22. Buy beautiful flowers for someone else.
23. Organize your space. Declutter.
24. Do shoulder rolls while at your computer.
25. Go to bed 8 hours before wakeup time.

SUCCESS TRACKER:

Bikini Body Checklist Week 12

☐ I've had foods that will help flatten my tummy and steered clear of foods that make me bloated.

☐ I've tried at least one belly-flattening recipe.

☐ I've packed my beach bag with all the must-have items that will keep me healthy and feeling good.

☐ I've followed the Bikini Diet meal plan.

☐ I've followed the Hot & Healthy Workout plan.

☐ I've made my very own Bliss List that I can turn to whenever I need to add some joy to my day.

Week 12 Measurements

Weight_____

Waist_____

Chest_____

Hips_____

This week I feel _____

_____

_____

_____

_____

_____

_____

_____

_____

_____

_____

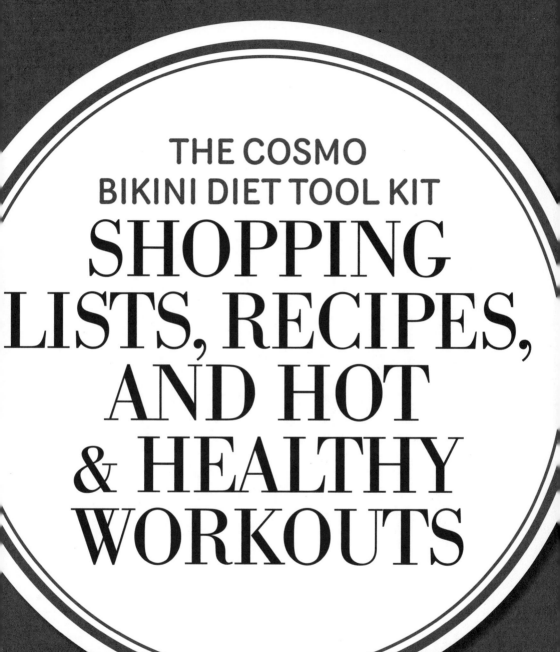

THE COSMO
BIKINI DIET TOOL KIT
SHOPPING LISTS, RECIPES, AND HOT & HEALTHY WORKOUTS

CHAPTER THIRTEEN

THE COSMO BIKINI DIET FOOD SHOPPING LISTS

NO MORE STRESSING OVER WHAT TO BUY AT THE GROCERY STORE!

Simply stock up on the food staples in the shopping list, and you'll always have nutritious, Bikini Diet–friendly options on hand. Then we've broken out the additional foods you'll need each week of the Bikini Diet. After you've finished the diet, keep the lists as a guide to keep your refrigerator and cupboards stocked with the healthy staples you'll always enjoy.

CORE BIKINI DIET SHOPPING LIST

BAKING STAPLES AND SPICES

Sesame oil	Pepper	Garlic powder
Extra-virgin olive oil	Cinnamon	Ginger
Cooking spray	Chili powder	Sugar or natural sugar
Dark chocolate chips	Cilantro	substitute such as stevia
Shredded coconut	Coriander	Nutmeg
Honey	Cumin	Parsley, dried
Maple syrup	Dill	Sweet paprika
Sea salt	Garlic	

BEVERAGES

Coffee	Tea
Milk	Seltzer water

BREADS

Whole wheat English muffins	Whole wheat pita	Whole wheat bread
	Whole wheat flatbread	

CANNED FOODS AND BOTTLED SAUCES

Black beans	Chicken stock	Light mayonnaise
Canned tuna	Mustard	Balsamic vinegar
Chickpeas	Light coconut milk	Worcestershire sauce

CEREAL AND GRAINS

Rolled oats	Low-fat granola	Quinoa
Whole grain cereal	Brown rice	

DAIRY, EGGS, REFRIGERATED FOODS

Reduced-fat Cheddar cheese	Laughing Cow cheese spread	Eggs
Low-fat cottage cheese	Parmesan cheese	Hummus
Part-skim mozzarella cheese sticks	Fat-free plain Greek yogurt	Low-fat milk
		Almond milk
		Orange juice

FRUIT AND VEGETABLES

Since produce can go bad quickly, just map out your weekly meal plan in advance and plan ahead for what you'll need that week so food doesn't go to waste. The following are included in at least one of the monthly meal plans.

Apples	Pineapple*	Onion (white and red)
Bananas	Asparagus	Red bell pepper
Berries: blueberries,	Avocado	Romaine lettuce
strawberries, and rasp-	Broccoli*	Spinach
berries*	Carrots*	Sweet potatoes
Grapes	Celery	Tomatoes
Lemon juice and lemons	Cucumber	Zucchini
Mango	Guacamole: 100-calorie	*CONSIDER BUYING
Pears	packs	THESE FROZEN

FROZEN FOODS

Frozen fruit and veggies	Veggie burgers	Whole grain waffles

MEAT, POULTRY, AND FISH

Chicken

NUTS, SEEDS, AND DRIED FRUIT

Almond butter	Raisins	Walnuts
Peanut butter	Pistachios	Macadamia nuts
Dried cranberries	Almonds	Chia seeds
Dried apricots	Cashews	Sunflower seeds

SNACK FOODS

Popcorn kernels (the	Whole grain baked	Whole wheat pretzels
kind for air popping)	tortilla chips	Whole wheat crackers
Salsa		

BIKINI DIET SHOPPING LIST

In addition to the core Bikini Diet shopping list above, grab these foods for this month's recipes.

BAKING STAPLES AND SPICES

All-purpose flour (can also substitute for whole-wheat flour)	Cayenne pepper Dark Chocolate Lemon pepper	White pepper

CANNED FOODS AND BOTTLED SAUCES

Apple sauce	Canned soup	Green olives

CEREAL AND GRAINS

Couscous

DAIRY, EGGS AND REFRIGERATED FOODS

Crumbled blue cheese Swiss cheese slices	Greek yogurt	Vanilla yogurt

FRUIT, VEGETABLES, AND HERBS

Cauliflower Green beans	Shallots Cherry tomatoes	Kiwi fruit

MEAT, POULTRY, AND FISH

Filet mignon or flank steak	Salmon

BIKINI DIET SHOPPING LIST

WEEKS
5-8

In addition to the core Bikini Diet shopping list,
grab these foods for this month's recipes.

BEVERAGES

Orange juice

CANNED FOODS AND BOTTLED SAUCES

Asian sesame vinaigrette
Black bean soup

Coconut milk
Light soy sauce

Teriyaki sauce

DAIRY, EGGS, AND REFIGERATED FOODS

Blueberry Greek yogurt

Strawberry Greek yogurt

FROZEN FOODS

Pint or single serve
light ice cream

Vegetable pot stickers/
frozen dumplings

FRUIT, VEGETABLES, AND HERBS

Edamame (shelled)
Jalapeño pepper
Mango

Scallions
Snow peas
Peaches

Mandarin oranges
Pineapple

MEAT, POULTRY AND FISH

Pork tenderloin

Tilapia filets
Mahi mahi filet

Sliced turkey breast

NUTS, SEEDS, AND DRIED FRUIT

Dry roasted edamame

Sesame seeds

PASTA

Soba noodles

SNACK FOODS

Salsa

BIKINI DIET SHOPPING LIST

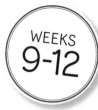

WEEKS
9-12

In addition to the core Bikini Diet shopping list,
grab these foods for this month's recipes.

BEVERAGES
Green tea

CANNED FOODS AND BOTTLED SAUCES
Black or kalamata olives	Nutella	Thousand Island
Canned soup	Pickles	dressing

CEREAL AND GRAINS
All-Bran cereal	Kashi 7-grain Puffs	Wild rice

DAIRY FOODS
Dark chocolate	Feta cheese	Strawberry-banana
almond milk		Greek yogurt

FRUIT, VEGETABLES, AND HERBS
Basil	Corn	Peaches
Butternut squash	Lime juice	Pineapple
Cherry tomatoes	Oranges	

MEAT, POULTRY, AND FISH
Flank steak	Lean ground beef and/or	Tuna steak
	ground sirlion	

NUTS, SEEDS, AND DRIED FRUIT
Dates or figs	Dried chopped apples	Pecans

CHAPTER FOURTEEN

QUICK & EASY BIKINI DIET RECIPES

READY, SET, COOK!

Now that you've stocked your kitchen with all the Bikini Diet staples you'll need to succeed, it's time to feed your taste buds. Here are all the recipes and meals for the Cosmo Bikini Diet, week by week. Remember: Day 7 of every week is your earned day for sticking to the healthy eating and fitness plan that week. (See page 34 on How to Plan Your Earned Day.) If you don't want to design your earned day, simply repeat one of the meals from the previous week's meal plan, but also allow yourself an extra treat.

RECIPES & MEALS

WEEKS
1-4

Breakfast

Day 1

¾ **cup Kashi GoLean Cereal** (or any cereal with less than 150 calories per cup, at least 5 grams of fiber, and less than 10 grams of sugar) with ½ ounce sliced almonds (11 almonds); ½ cup low-fat or almond milk, and ½ cup sliced strawberries (or other berries like raspberries, blackberries, or blueberries)

Coffee or tea (black or with 1 teaspoon added sugar or sugar substitute)

Day 2

1 egg scrambled: Scramble your egg the Bikini Diet way with a light spray of olive oil (¼ teaspoon) in a skillet. Sauté over medium heat for 3 minutes or until the egg is fully cooked. Serve with 1 slice of 100% whole-wheat bread, toasted.

Have a side of **½ cup of raspberries** (or blackberries, blueberries, or strawberries)

Coffee or tea (black or with 1 teaspoon added sugar or sugar substitute)

Day 3

Whole wheat English muffin, toasted and topped with 1 wedge cheese spread (like Laughing Cow Original Swiss Cheese Spread) and 1 cup blackberries

Coffee or tea (black or with 1 teaspoon added sugar or sugar substitute)

Day 4

APPLE CINNAMON OATMEAL

Prepare or warm ½ cup slow-cooked oats or other hot whole-grain cereal (such as Bob's Red Mill). Top it with ½ cup sliced apples, 1 teaspoon maple syrup and ¼ teaspoon cinnamon.

Coffee or tea (black or with 1 teaspoon added sugar or sugar substitute)

Day 5

1 whole wheat waffle (such as Eggo Nutri-Grain Waffles with 90 calories per waffle or a similar kind) topped with 2 teaspoons nut butter (like almond or peanut butter) and 1 small banana, sliced

Coffee or tea (black or with 1 teaspoon added sugar or sugar substitute)

Day 6

MEXICAN BREAKFAST SCRAMBLE

◆ Sauté ¼ cup chopped red bell peppers and ¼ cup chopped sweet onion in a small pan for 5 to 7 minutes or until tender. Add ½ cup salsa and 2 eggs (beaten), scramble until cooked well. Serve with 1 tablespoon plain Greek yogurt.

Coffee or tea (black or with 1 teaspoon added sugar or sugar substitute)

Lunch

Day 1

TUNA FISH SALAD SANDWICH

◆ Combine 5-ounce can of tuna (drained) with 1 stalk celery (chopped), 1 teaspoon olive oil, 2 tablespoons lemon juice, and salt and pepper to taste
◆ To make the tuna fish sandwich, take 2 slices of whole wheat bread and fill with 4 ounces (about ½ cup) tuna plus romaine lettuce and a slice of tomato.

Apple

Seltzer water

Day 2

Large bowl (1 ½ cups) black bean and vegetable soup, such as Health Valley or similar kind with 120 calories per cup

2 slices of bread, or whole-wheat baguette that's about 1 ounce (28 grams) with 110 calories or less

1 large apple with ¾ ounce Baybel or similar cheese

Unsweetened tea

Day 3

CHICKEN & VEGGIE WRAP

◆ Fill a 100-calorie whole-wheat wrap (like Flatout Light Wraps) with 3 ounces pulled chicken tagine (left over from dinner on Day 1) or grilled chicken and ½ cup baby spinach. Drizzle with remaining marinade or Healthy Balsamic Dressing (see recipe on page 165).

SPINACH SALAD

◆ 1 cup baby spinach topped with 1 cup chopped vegetables (any type) with **Healthy Balsamic Dressing** (see page 165)
TIP: In place of making the Healthy Balsamic Dressing, you can opt for a store-bought light balsamic that's about 100 calories or less per serving.

Seltzer water

HEALTHY BALSAMIC DRESSING

Courtesy of Jonathan Rollo, chef and owner Greenleaf Gourmet Chopshop in Los Angeles.

(SERVES 32, 1 TABLESPOON PER SERVING)

INGREDIENTS

½ red onion, chopped
1 shallot, chopped
2 cloves of garlic, chopped
1 cup olive oil plus 1 tablespoon
1 avocado
1 tablespoon sugar
1 cup balsamic vinegar
¼ cup Worcestershire sauce

DIRECTIONS

◆ In sauté pan, slightly brown chopped onion, shallot, and garlic with 1 tablespoon of olive oil. Remove and cool. Add all ingredients to blender except the remaining oil. Begin to blend and drizzle oil slowly into mixture to emulsify and make it creamy. Store in glass jar in refrigerator.

Day 4

VEGGIE PITA

◆ Open a whole-wheat pita so there are two pockets to fill. Spread each half with 1 tablespoon of hummus. Then fill both halves with ½ cup dark leafy greens (like romaine) and ¼ cup chopped vegetables (any variety will work great). Finish with a slice of 50% reduced-fat Cheddar (about 1 ounce) split between the two halves.

½ cup cottage cheese topped with ½ cup cubed pineapple

Seltzer water

Day 5

ITALIAN FLATBREAD

◆ On a round flatbread (like Arnolds whole-wheat flatbread), add ½ cup baby spinach and 3 ounces sliced grilled chicken. Top with 2 tablespoons balsamic dressing. *Look for varieties with 100 calories or less, like Wishbone Balsamic and Basil Vinaigrette, or use 1 tablespoon of the Healthy Balsamic Dressing from the lunch recipe on Day 3.

Tomatoes: 5 cherry tomatoes

Fruit: 1 piece of fruit of your choice (e.g. apple, pear, banana, orange, or ½ cup grapes or berries)

Water or seltzer water

Day 6

VEGGIE & CHICKEN SALAD

Fill a bowl with 2 cups dark leafy greens (like romaine or baby spinach); 1 cup chopped vegetables (any variety); 3 ounces protein (tuna salad, leftover chicken, or sliced steak). Serve with 1 tablespoon Healthy Balsamic dressing (or 1 teaspoon olive oil and 1 teaspoon balsamic vinegar)

6 ounces Greek yogurt topped with ½ cup grapes

Seltzer water

Dinner

Day 1

CHICKEN TAGINE WITH OLIVES

(SERVES 4)

INGREDIENTS

¼ cup olive oil, plus 2 tablespoons
1 teaspoon cumin*
1 teaspoon coriander*
1 teaspoon sweet paprika*
½ teaspoon cinnamon*
¼ teaspoon ground ginger*
1 4-pound chicken, cut into 8 pieces
   (or 4 chicken breasts)
1 teaspoon salt
¼ teaspoon freshly ground black pepper*
2 onions, thinly sliced
1 garlic clove, minced
½ cup pitted green olives
1½ cups chicken stock
2 tablespoons minced fresh cilantro
   (or 2 teaspoons dried cilantro)
2 tablespoons minced fresh flat-leaf
parsley (or 2 teaspoons dried parsley)
Juice and zest of 1 lemon or 3 tablespoons
   lemon juice

TIP: Instead of stocking up on tons of spices, try McCormick's Recipe Inspirations Chicken Tikka Masala which has paprika, garlic, black pepper, coriander, cumin, cinnamon, and red pepper.

DIRECTIONS

◆ In a large bowl, combine ¼ cup olive oil, cumin, coriander, paprika, cinnamon, and ginger.

◆ Season chicken with salt and pepper, and add to marinade. Stir until marinade covers each piece. Refrigerate at least 2 hours or up to 24 hours.

◆ Take chicken out of marinade, and pat dry. Reserve marinade.

◆ Heat 2 tablespoons olive oil in a heavy-bottom stockpot. Brown chicken, skin-side down, 4 to 5 minutes. Turn, and brown an additional 3 to 4 minutes. Remove chicken, and put on a plate.

◆ Add onions and garlic to the stockpot, and sauté until tender, about 5 minutes. Add reserved marinade and chicken, green olives, stock, and additional salt and pepper. Bring to a low boil, and reduce heat to a simmer. Cover, and cook 45 minutes.

◆ Stir in cilantro, parsley, lemon juice, and lemon zest. Serve with pita to soak up any remaining sauce.

APRICOT-HERB COUSCOUS

(SERVES 6)

INGREDIENTS

1 10-ounce box couscous
¼ cup minced fresh flat-leaf parsley
¼ cup chopped dried apricots
¼ cup shaved almonds
1 tablespoon extra-virgin olive oil
1 tablespoon fresh lemon juice
Salt and pepper

DIRECTIONS

◆ Prepare couscous to package instructions. Stir in parsley, apricots, almonds, olive oil, and lemon juice. Season with salt and pepper.

STEAMED ASPARAGUS

◆ Prepare 7 asparagus spears per serving. Trim the tough part off of the bottom of the asparagus, place in a skillet with enough water to cover the bottom of the pan (but not completely covering the asparagus). Over medium heat, bring water to a boil and then cover. Simmer for 3 minutes. Drain and serve tossed with lemon juice and garlic powder (to taste).

1 cup of milk or milk substitute

TIP: Make Your Own Microwave Meal: If you have leftovers from this meal, portion ½ cup of Apricot-Herb Couscous and 7 asparagus spears in a single-serve container and freeze for another night when you're short on time.

Day 2

FLANK STEAK OR FILET MIGNON WITH SAUTÉED ONIONS

(SERVES 2)

◆ Place two 4-ounce filet mignon or flank steak fillets on the broiler pan in oven, then put under the broiler for 5 minutes. Turn the filets, and broil for 5 minutes more (or until desired doneness).

◆ While the meat is broiling, sauté 1 sweet onion sliced thin in a skillet with 1 teaspoon of extra virgin olive oil until tender, about 5 minutes. Serve one filet topped with ½ the sautéed onion.

TIP: Save the remaining filet and onion for a dinner later in the week!

BAKED SWEET POTATO

◆ Scrub a small sweet potato (about 4-inches in length), and then pierce with a fork several times. Microwave the sweet potato for 5 minutes, transfer to the oven, and bake at 350 degrees for 20 minutes. Top with a drizzle (1 teaspoon) of maple syrup before serving.

TIP: If you skip the microwave step, bake for 60 minutes, or until tender.

STEAMED GREEN BEANS

◆ Steam or microwave 1 cup green beans until tender. Season with salt and pepper to taste.

TIP: Frozen green beans work great!

1 cup milk or milk substitute

Day 3

VEGGIE-AVOCADO BURGER ON TOMATO BUN

◆ Prepare a veggie burger (like Amy's Kitchen All American Veggie Burger). Top and serve it with ¼ of an avocado, sliced, between two thick slices of tomatoes. Drizzle with mustard.

Pineapple: ½ cup fresh cubed pineapple

SAUTÉED ZUCCHINI

◆ Thinly slice one small zucchini (about 1 cup). In a sauté pan, add 1 teaspoon olive oil, then add the sliced zucchini. Sauté for 5 to 7 minutes or until tender. Sprinkle with ½ teaspoon garlic powder and serve.

1 cup milk or milk substitute

Day 4

STEAK SALAD

◆ Fill a bowl with 2 cups dark greens, like romaine lettuce; add 1 cup chopped veggies of your choice (such as red bell pepper, cucumbers, or carrots), and top with 4 ounces of the leftover broiled filet mignon or flank steak from Day 2 dinner, sliced, with the remaining ½ cup sautéed onions. Finish with 2 tablespoons crumbled blue cheese.

GARLIC TOAST

◆ Toast a slice of whole-wheat bread with ½ teaspoon olive oil and garlic powder to taste (about ¼ teaspoon). Toast under the broiler (about 1 minute) until bread is lightly toasted.

1 cup milk or milk substitute

Day 5

GRILLED SALMON

◆ Grill or broil 5 ounces wild salmon (cooks down to about 4 ounces) for about 6 to 8 minutes per side or until cooked through. Season with ¼ teaspoon lemon pepper before serving.

MASHED CAULIFLOWER

◆ Microwave or steam cauliflower until tender. Then mash with a fork, season with white pepper and a dash of sea salt for flavor.

½ cup sliced mango

1 cup milk or milk substitute

Day 6

CHEESY TOMATO WRAP

◆ Top a 100-calorie flatbread with 2 slices Swiss cheese and 1 sliced plum tomato. Place in oven at 350 degrees for 3 to 5 minutes or until the cheese is melted. Wrap up and serve.

1 cup butternut squash soup (like Amy's Organic Butternut Squash Soup, or a similar type with 100-120 calories and 340 milligrams of sodium or less per serving)

1 cup milk or milk substitute

Snacks & Desserts

Day 1

½ cup sliced cucumbers (or other veggies like red peppers, cherry tomatoes or baby carrots) with 2 teaspoons hummus

½ cup Greek yogurt topped with 1 teaspoon of honey and ½ ounce almonds (11 almonds)

Flex Calories: 150 calories to spend however you choose, such as on a glass of wine or a few squares of dark chocolate. Remember: Flex Calories kick in on Week 2 following the Jump-Start Week.

Day 2

POPCORN WITH SPICE & SALT

1 cup air-popped popcorn with a sprinkle of cayenne pepper, sea salt, and 1 tablespoon grated Parmesan cheese

½ cup low-fat cottage cheese with 1 sliced kiwi fruit

Flex Calories: 150 calories to spend however you choose

Day 3

2 small squares dark chocolate with ½ cup sliced strawberries

¼ cup dried apricots and 1 tablespoon sunflower seeds (hulled variety, with shells removed)

Flex Calories: 150 calories to spend however you choose

Day 4

100-calorie pack of guacamole (like Wholly Guacamole single-serve packs) with ½ cup veggies for dipping (red bell pepper, cucumbers, or celery)

Part-skim or reduced-fat cheese stick (1 ounce) and a pear

Flex Calories: 150 calories to spend however you choose

Day 5

1 large hard-boiled egg with 10 wheat crackers (such as Kashi Honey Sesame Crackers or similar cracker with 80 calories)

24 pistachios (with the shell, so they take longer to eat) and ¼ cup dried cranberries

BERRIES WITH VANILLA YOGURT

For dessert, have ½ cup mango with 1 tablespoon Greek vanilla yogurt, or skip it and spend **150 Flex Calories** however you choose.

Day 6

½ cup applesauce

½ ounce almonds (11 almonds)

1 celery stalk filled with 1 tablespoon or peanut butter or nut butter and topped with 1 tablespoon raisins

Flex Calories: 150 calories to spend however you choose

WEEKLY AVERAGE DAILY NUTRITION FACTS: About 1500 calories plus 150 Flex Calories for about 1,650 calories total, 53 grams total fat, 15 grams saturated fat, 0 grams trans fat, 17 grams monounsaturated fat, 6 grams polyunsaturated fat, 242 milligrams cholesterol, 2,148 milligrams sodium, 174 grams carbohydrates, 30 grams fiber, 74 grams sugar, 90 grams protein. Ratio of calories from carbohydrates, protein, and fat: 50% carbohydrates, 23% protein, and 27% fat.

RECIPES & MEALS

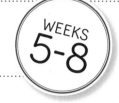

WEEKS
5-8

Breakfast

Day 1

WAFFLE & EGGS
◆ Toast one whole-grain frozen waffle (like Lifestream Flax Plus Waffles), and top it with one scrambled egg

1 cup of raspberries or other fruit

Coffee or tea (black or with 1 teaspoon added sugar or sugar substitute)

Day 2

COTTAGE CHEESE & BERRIES:
◆ 1 cup of low-fat cottage cheese topped with ½ cup blueberries (or other berries)

Coffee or tea (black or with 1 teaspoon added sugar or sugar substitute)

Day 3

BLUEBERRY CHIA SMOOTHIE
◆ In a blender combine 6 ounces nonfat blueberry Greek yogurt; ¾ cup frozen blueberries; 1 teaspoon chia seeds; and ¼ cup low fat milk or milk substitute. Blend until smooth and serve immediately.

Coffee or tea (black or with 1 teaspoon added sugar or sugar substitute)

Day 4

MANGO-COCONUT OATMEAL
◆ Prepare or warm ½ cup rolled oats and top with ½ cup diced mango, 1 tablespoon of shredded coconut, and ¼ cup light coconut milk or milk

Coffee or tea (black or with 1 teaspoon added sugar or sugar substitute)

Day 5

AVOCADO SMOOTHIE
Courtesy Fernando Coppola, executive chef, W Retreat & Spa, Vieques Island
◆ In a blender with a handful of ice, combine ¼ avocado (pit and skin removed), 4 strawberries (frozen or fresh), and 1 cup orange juice. Blend until smooth. Serve immediately.

½ ounce almonds (11 almonds)

Coffee or tea (black or with 1 teaspoon added sugar or sugar substitute)

Day 6

EGGS & SPINACH SCRAMBLED ON TOAST

◆ Sauté 1 cup of spinach with 1 teaspoon of olive oil until wilted, about 3 minutes. Then add in one large egg, scramble until cooked through. Season with salt and pepper. Serve on 1 slice of 100% whole wheat toast

Coffee or tea (black or with 1 teaspoon added sugar or sugar substitute)

Lunch

Day 1

ALMOND BUTTER AND PEAR SANDWICH

◆ On one slice of whole-wheat bread, spread 1 tablespoon almond butter (½ a golf ball's worth) and top it with one sliced pear

½ cup dry-roasted edamame

½ cup red bell pepper slices with ¼ cup hummus

Seltzer water

Day 2

TURKEY SUB

◆ Order a 6" turkey sub (e.g. Subway) or whole-wheat roll with all the veggie toppings and honey mustard dressing OR make your own turkey sandwich with 2 ounces sliced turkey breast on 2 slices 100% whole wheat bread topped with sliced

cucumbers, tomatoes, and lettuce and a drizzle (1 teaspoon) honey mustard.

½ cup carrots (sliced) with 2 tablespoons hummus

½ cup grapes

Seltzer water

Day 3

1 cup black bean soup (like Amy's Organic Black Bean Vegetable Soup, or similar soup with 120-140 calories or less per serving)

8 whole-wheat crackers (like Triscuit or Kashi Roasted Garlic Crackers) with 8 thin slices (1 ½ ounces) low-fat Cheddar cheese (like Cabot 50% light cheese)

Medium apple

Seltzer water

Day 4

HUMMUS AND CUCUMBER PITA SANDWICH

◆ Fill two whole-wheat pita halves (1 pita) each with 2 tablespoons hummus, ¼ cup cucumber slices, ½ ounce reduced-fat cheese (like Cabot 50% Light Cheddar) and a drizzle of honey mustard (about 1 teaspoon or less)

½ cup sliced strawberries

Seltzer water

Day 5
THAI CHOPPED CHICKEN SALAD

(SERVES 1)

INGREDIENTS

2 cups romaine lettuce
4 ounces grilled chicken breast, sliced
¼ cup mandarin oranges, drained
¼ cup sliced cucumbers
1 tablespoon sesame seeds
3 tablespoons slivered almonds
2 tablespoons Asian sesame vinaigrette
(Such as Wishbone Asian Sesame &
Ginger Vinaigrette or another type with
70 calories per 2 tablespoons)

DIRECTIONS

◆ Fill a bowl with romaine lettuce. Top
with the grilled chicken, mandarin oranges, cucumbers, sesame seeds, and almonds.
◆ Toss with the vinaigrette or serve on
the side.

TIP: If preparing to take with you on the
go, leave the vinaigrette on the side so the
salad does not get soggy!

Medium apple

Unsweetened tea

Day 6

BREAKFAST FOR LUNCH! CRANBERRY CRUNCH YOGURT PARFAIT

◆ In a bowl or to-go container if bringing
to work, layer 6 ounces yogurt (¾ cup),
½ ounce cashews, ¼ cup dried cranberries,
and ¼ cup granola.

Seltzer water

Dinner

Day 1

MACADAMIA-CRUSTED TILAPIA FILLET TOPPED WITH PINEAPPLE SALSA

(SERVES 2)

INGREDIENTS

For fish:
¼ cup all-purpose flour
1 egg, lightly beaten
¼ cup crushed macadamia nuts
2 tilapia fillets (about 3 to 4 ounces each)

For salsa:
1 cup finely chopped fresh pineapple
1 tablespoon minced red onion
½ jalapeño, seeds removed, minced
¼ cup minced cilantro
Salt and pepper

DIRECTIONS

◆ Preheat oven to 400 degrees. Put flour,
egg, and nuts in three separate shallow
dishes. Dredge each fillet first in flour, then
egg, then nuts.
◆ Place on oiled baking sheet. Bake 12 to
14 minutes or until golden brown.
The fish is done when it is opaque and
flakes easily with a fork.
◆ While fish is baking, make the salsa.
Combine pineapple, onion, jalapeño, and
cilantro. Season with salt and pepper.
Serve with fish.

SPEEDY SESAME SNOW PEAS

(SERVES 2)

INGREDIENTS

1 cup snow peas
1 teaspoon unsalted butter or olive oil
½ teaspoon sesame seeds
Salt and pepper

DIRECTIONS

◆ Rinse snow peas but don't dry. Place in a microwavable bowl, and microwave on high for 45 seconds. Stir in butter, sesame seeds, and salt and pepper.

TIP: Save the leftovers for a meal later in the week.

1 cup milk or milk substitute

Day 2

Wonton Soup
1 cup wonton soup (look for 100-120 calories per cup, like Annie Chan's Chicken and Cilantro Wonton Soup!)

SOBA NOODLE BOWL

◆ In a skillet, combine 1 cup sliced zucchini, ½ cup shelled edamame (soybeans), and sauté with ½ teaspoon sesame oil until the zucchini are tender, about 5 minutes. Add ½ cup cooked soba noodles and 1 tablespoon teriyaki sauce. Sauté until the noodles and sauce are combined with the vegetables and warmed.

1 cup milk or milk substitute

Day 3

GRILLED PORK TENDERLOIN WITH ROASTED GRAPES

(SERVES 4)

INGREDIENTS

½ teaspoons cracked black pepper
2 teaspoons extra virgin olive oil
1-pound pork tenderloin
3 cups grapes
½ cup water

DIRECTIONS

◆ Preheat oven to 475 degrees. Rub the pork with cracked black pepper. In a skillet with an oven-safe handle, heat oil over medium heat. Add pork and cook for 5 minutes, turning to brown on all sides.

◆ Add grapes and ½ cup of water. Cover, and put in oven to roast for about 15 minutes or until meat thermometer reaches 150 degrees.

◆ Transfer pork to platter and slice. Heat the grape mixture to boiling over high heat boil until liquid thickens, and then pour over sliced pork.

½ cup leftover Speedy Sesame Snow Peas from Day 1

½ cup cooked brown rice with a sprinkle of garlic powder and salt to taste

Day 4

TROPICAL MAHI MAHI SALAD

◆ Grill or broil one 5-ounce mahi mahi filet until cooked throughout, about 8 to 10 minutes per side.

◆ Fill a bowl with 2 cups of dark leafy greens (any type, such as romaine, spinach, or arugula). Top the salad with the cooked and sliced mahi mahi filet; 1 cup chopped vegetables (sliced red bell pepper, cucumbers, cherry tomatoes) and toss with 2 tablespoons Asian sesame salad dressing (such as Wishbone Light Asian Sesame & Ginger Vinaigrette or similar kind with 70 calories per 2 tablespoons or less)

BAKED SWEET POTATO

◆ Scrub a small sweet potato (about 4 inches in length), and then pierce with a fork several times. Microwave the sweet potato for 5 minutes. Then transfer to the oven and bake at 350 degrees for 20 minutes. Top with a drizzle (1 teaspoon) of maple syrup before serving.

TIP: If you skip the microwave step, bake for 60 minutes or until tender.

1 cup milk or milk substitute

Day 5

POT STICKERS WITH GINGER-LEMON DIPPING SAUCE

(SERVES 3; 4 DUMPLINGS EACH)

INGREDIENTS

3 tablespoons light soy sauce

2 tablespoons freshly-squeezed lemon juice

1 teaspoon fresh ginger, grated, (or ¼ teaspoon ground ginger)

1 teaspoon toasted sesame oil

1 scallion, thinly sliced

12 frozen dumplings

DIRECTIONS

◆ Buy frozen dumplings (shrimp, chicken, pork, or vegetable, like Health is Wealth Veggie Potstickers) and cook according to package instructions.

◆ In a small dish, combine soy sauce, lemon juice, ginger, oil, and scallion to dip with dumplings.

ASIAN VEGETABLES

◆ In a skillet or wok, add 2 cups Asian stir-fry vegetables (broccoli, snow peas, red pepper slices, yellow pepper slices), and sauté with 1 teaspoon sesame oil, 1 teaspoon of light soy sauce and ½ teaspoon each ground ginger and garlic powder. Sauté until vegetables are tender, about 3 to 5 minutes. Serve with pot stickers.

EDAMAME

◆ Steam or microwave 1 cup fresh or frozen edamame for 3 minutes or until tender.

1 cup milk or milk substitute

Day 6
FLATBREAD ASPARAGUS PIZZA
◆ First steam or microwave 7 spears asparagus until tender. Then, on flatbread, drizzle 1 teaspoon of olive oil and top it with 2 chopped spears (save the rest to eat with the meal) and ¼ cup shredded low-fat Cheddar cheese (like Cabot 50% Light Cheddar Cheese). Place in a 350 degrees oven for 10 minutes or until cheese is melted.

STRAWBERRY SPINACH SALAD
◆ Top 1 cup baby spinach with ¼ cup sliced strawberries, 2 teaspoons chopped walnuts, and 1 tablespoon Healthy Balsamic Dressing (See recipe on page 165).

1 cup milk or milk substitute

Snacks & Desserts

Day 1
TURKEY AND CHEESE ROLL-UPS
◆ Take 2 slices (about 2 ounces) oven-roasted turkey breast (like Boar's Head), and spread each with a Laughing Cow spreadable cheese wedge. Then roll it up. If you're on the go, place the roll-ups in a baggie to make them portable, and store in your fridge at work.

CHIPS WITH SALSA
◆ ¼ cup salsa and 1 ounce (small handful) whole-grain tortilla chips (like Guiltless Gourmet or other chips with 110 calories or less per serving and 2 grams of fat or less)

150 Flex Calories to spend however you choose

Day 2
1 hard-boiled egg with medium apple

1 small banana, sliced. Top each slice with a light spread of peanut butter (2 teaspoons peanut butter) or other nut butter (e.g. almond butter)

150 Flex Calories to spend however you choose. Have a glass of wine, a small dessert, or add in an extra snack!

Day 3
¼ raisins and ½ ounce peanuts

¼ cup of tuna salad (See recipe on Week 1, page 164) and ½ cup celery

STRAWBERRY WAFFLE SUNDAE DESSERT
◆ Toast 1 whole grain waffle, and top with ½ cup sliced strawberries and 1 tablespoon strawberry Greek yogurt. Or skip it and spend **150 Flex Calories** however you choose.

Day 4

1 medium apple, sliced, with 2 teaspoons almond butter or other nut butter

CHIA SEED PUDDING

(SERVES 5, ½-CUP SERVINGS)

INGREDIENTS

½ cup chia seeds
2 cups almond milk
2 tablespoons pure maple syrup

DIRECTIONS

Add all ingredients in an air-tight container, and stir to combine. Store in the refrigerator overnight. Serve the next day topped with a sprinkle of cinnamon. Note: The chia seeds expand by absorbing the almond milk, so the texture will thicken as it sits overnight.

150 Flex Calories to spend however you choose.

Day 5

4 whole-wheat crackers (like Triscuit or Kashi Roasted Garlic Crackers) with 1 ounce of sliced reduced-fat Cheddar cheese (about 4 dice-size cubes)

½ cup whole-grain cereal (like Barbara's Bakery Shredded Spoonfuls or similar cereal with 80 calories per ½ cup and at least 3 grams of fiber) with ¼ cup milk and 1 small banana, sliced

150 Flex Calories to spend however you choose.

Day 6

½ cup sliced red bell peppers, 4 whole wheat pretzel sticks with 4 ounces (½ cup) plain Greek yogurt, seasoned with 1 teaspoon garlic powder and ¼ teaspoon dill

1 spreadable cheese wedge (like Laughing Cow Original, Swiss Creamy) and a pear

LIGHT ICE CREAM WITH FRUIT

◆ For dessert, have ½ cup light ice cream topped with ½ cup sliced peaches or other fruit of your choice. Or skip it and spend **150 Flex Calories** however you choose.

WEEKLY AVERAGE DAILY NUTRITION FACTS: About 1,500 calories plus 150 Flex Calories for about 1,650 calories total, 50 grams fat, 13 grams saturated fat, 0 grams trans fat 11 g monounsaturated fat, 5g polyunsaturated fat, 219 mg cholesterol, 2549 mg sodium, 193 g carbs, 30 g fiber, 80 grams of sugar, 85 g protein. Ratio of calories from carbohydrates, protein, and fat: 50% carbohydrates, 20% protein, and 30% fat

RECIPES & MEALS

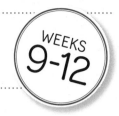

Breakfast

Day 1

WARM QUINOA, CHIA, & FRUIT CEREAL

◆ Combine ½ cup quinoa (cooked in almond milk), 1 tablespoon chia seeds, ½ cup peaches or berries, ¼ teaspoon cinnamon, ¼ teaspoon nutmeg (optional), and 1 teaspoon honey.

TIP: Make a large batch of quinoa and then have it ready to go for quick breakfasts all week long!

Coffee or tea (black or with 1 teaspoon added sugar or sugar substitute)

Day 2

SLIM MIXER

◆ Combine ½ cup Smart Bran Original or All-Bran cereal (or similar cereal with at least 10 grams of fiber per ½ cup); 1 cup puffed kamut or Kashi 7 Whole Grain Puffs cereal (or similar cereal with 70 calories per cup and 0 grams of sugar); 1 cup vanilla almond milk; and ½ cup berries.

Coffee or tea (black or with 1 teaspoon added sugar or sugar substitute)

Day 3

VEGGIE & EGG MELT

◆ Scramble one whole egg with ½ cup of baby spinach over medium heat until cooked thoroughly. Top with 3 tablespoons of shredded light Cheddar cheese (like Cabot 50% Light Cheddar cheese). Place on half whole-wheat English muffin and top with one slice of tomato.

One orange

Coffee or tea (black or with 1 teaspoon added sugar or sugar substitute)

Day 4

6 ounce cup of nonfat (any flavor) Greek yogurt and ½ ounce almonds (11 almonds)

Coffee or tea (black or with 1 teaspoon added sugar or sugar substitute)

Day 5
MANGO SMOOTHIE
◆ In a blender, combine 6 ounces plain or mango-flavored Greek yogurt, 1 cup sliced mango (fresh or frozen), 2 teaspoons honey, and ¼ cup milk or almond milk. Blend until smooth.

Coffee or tea (black or with 1 teaspoon added sugar or sugar substitute)

Day 6
TOMATO & CHEESE OATMEAL
◆ Top cooked oatmeal with ¼ cup shredded Cheddar cheese (reduced fat or 2% light), 1 tablespoon diced red onion, and ¼ cup diced tomato.

Coffee or tea (black or with 1 teaspoon added sugar or sugar substitute)

Lunch

Day 1
MEDITERRANEAN CHOPPED SALAD
(SERVES 1)

INGREDIENTS
¾ cup canned chickpeas, drained and rinsed
2 cups total chopped cucumbers, tomatoes, and yellow bell peppers
1 to 2 tablespoons chopped fresh basil and parsley (optional)
1 teaspoon olive oil
2 tablespoons fresh lemon juice
Pinch of salt
½ cup cooled cooked quinoa

DIRECTIONS
◆ Combine all ingredients and serve.

½ cup grapes

Unsweetened tea

Day 2
GRILLED CHEESE & TOMATO SANDWICH
◆ Place two slices of whole-wheat bread on a baking sheet. Top each with two to three tomato slices and two ounces shredded Cheddar cheese (like Cabot 50% light Cheddar cheese).
◆ Place on a baking sheet or in a toaster oven and bake at 350 degrees for 5 to 7 minutes, or until the cheese is melted. Eat as two open-faced sandwiches or combine as one sandwich.

½ cup cucumber slices with 2 tablespoons hummus

1 piece of fruit (apple, banana, orange, pear, or ½ cup of berries or grapes)

Seltzer water

Day 3
TACO SALAD BOWL
◆ Saute ¼ cup each sliced peppers and onions with 1 teaspoon olive oil for 5 to 7 minutes until tender.
◆ Mix 2 cups romaine lettuce, 4 ounces diced grilled chicken, ½ cup black beans, ½ cup sautéed peppers and onions*, ¼ cup salsa, 2 tablespoons plain Greek yogurt, and ¼ cup corn.
 (Eat-out option is to order Chipotle's Taco Salad Bowl with romaine lettuce, grilled chicken, black beans, fajita vegetables, tomato salsa, and corn salsa)

Unsweetened iced tea

Day 4
COBB SALAD
◆ Fill a bowl with 2 cups shredded romaine lettuce. Then top with 1 hard-boiled egg, chopped; 5 cherry tomatoes; ½ cup black bean and corn salad (see recipe on page 183) and ¼ of an avocado sliced.
TIP: The black bean and corn salad doubles as the dressing!

Day 5
MEDITERRANEAN PLATTER
◆ On a platter or in a to-go-container, arrange 1 whole-wheat pita bread (sliced into triangles); ½ cup sliced red peppers; ½ cup sliced cucumbers; 6 black or Kalamata olives; ¼ cup crumbled feta cheese; 4 ounces plain Greek yogurt mixed with ¼ teaspoon dill and ¼ teaspoon garlic powder; and ¼ cup of hummus.
TIP: Opt for pita bread with about 140 calories or less

Unsweetened tea

Day 6
BREAKFAST FOR LUNCH! STRAWBERRY-BANANA PARFAIT
◆ In a dish or to-go container, alternate layers of 6 ounces strawberry-banana flavored Greek yogurt (like Chobani) with ½ cup total granola (like Nature's Path), and 1 small banana, sliced.

1 Medium pear

Seltzer water

Dinner

Day 1

BEEF BURGER LETTUCE WRAP

(SERVES 2)

INGREDIENTS

4-ounce lean grass-fed beef patty, cooked
2 large romaine or red-leaf lettuce leaves
Sliced pickles (1 ounce)
Sliced tomato
1 tablespoon Thousand Island dressing
(like Newman's Own)

DIRECTIONS

◆ Assemble your burger between the two lettuce leaves, and serve with the sides.

Hummus and crudités: Have a side of 1½ cup crudités (baby carrots, celery sticks, broccoli spears, etc.) with 1 tablespoon hummus

1 cup low-fat milk or milk substitute

Day 2

GRILLED CHILI-RUBBED FLANK STEAK

(SERVES 4)

INGREDIENTS

1 pound flank steak
1 tablespoon chili powder
1 teaspoon cumin
1 teaspoon coriander
Salt and pepper (optional)

DIRECTIONS

◆ Preheat a grill or grill pan to medium-high heat. In a small dish, combine chili powder, cumin, and coriander. Rub the spice mixture onto both sides of the steak. Season with salt and pepper (optional). Grill about 5 minutes per side. Transfer to a cutting board, and let rest about 5 minutes. Slice on the diagonal. Can be served hot, or refrigerate until serving.

BAKED SWEET POTATO

◆ Scrub a small sweet potato (about 4 inches in length), and then pierce with a fork several times. Microwave for 5 minutes. Then transfer to the oven and bake at 350 degrees for 20 minutes. Top with a drizzle (1 teaspoon) of maple syrup before serving.

TIP: If you skip the microwave step, bake for 60 minutes, or until tender.

Broccoli: Steam or microwave ½ cup of broccoli florets. Toss with lemon juice, garlic powder, and salt to taste.

1 cup low-fat milk or milk substitute

Day 3

BREAKFAST FOR DINNER! WAFFLES WITH BERRIES AND YOGURT

◆ Toast two whole-grain blueberry waffles (like Kashi Go Lean Blueberry Waffles or similar kind with 170 calories for 2 waffles, 6 grams of fiber and 4 grams of sugar or less). Top each with ½ cup mixed berries and ¼ cup plain Greek yogurt. Finish with a drizzle of 1 tablespoon of pure maple syrup.

ORANGE JUICE FREEZE

◆ In a blender, combine 1 cup of 100% orange juice with a handful of ice cubes. Blend until whipped and icy. Serve immediately.

Day 4

FLANK STEAK SANDWICH WITH PEPPERS AND ONIONS

◆ Prepare a 4-ounce portion of **Grilled Chili-Rubbed Flank Steak** (see recipe on page 180) Sauté ½ cup sliced sweet onions and ¼ cup of red bell pepper for 3 to 5 minutes, until tender. Then add 4 ounces sliced Chili-Rubbed Flank Steak and heat until warmed through. Toast a slice of whole-wheat bread with a ¼ teaspoon of garlic powder, then top it with the sliced flank steak and sautéed onions and peppers.

SWEET POTATO FRIES

◆ Slice a small sweet potato lengthwise into fries. Place on baking sheet and drizzle with 1 teaspoon olive oil. Bake in a 425-degree oven for 20 to 25 minutes until the fries are crispy.

ROASTED ASPARAGUS

◆ Wash and prepare asparagus by trimming off the tough bottom ends (about ½-inch). Add to the sweet potatoes and roast. After 15 minutes, remove the asparagus and set aside.

Unsweetened tea

Day 5

PAN-SEARED TUNA

◆ Heat a skillet over medium heat. Season a 4-ounce ahi or yellowfin tuna filet with cracked black pepper. Spray the pan with cooking spray or 1 teaspoon olive oil. Then place tuna filet on the skillet; cook for 4 minutes per side or until the tuna is done per your liking. Prepare the lime-avocado salsa by slicing ¼ of an avocado and tossing with 1 teaspoon lime juice and ¼ teaspoon garlic powder. Serve over the cooked tuna.

ROASTED BUTTERNUT SQUASH

◆ Take 1 cup cubed butternut squash (fresh or frozen) and place on a baking sheet. Roast in a 425-degree oven for 15 to 20 minutes (for fresh) or 30 to 35 minutes (for frozen), until lightly browned.

Lemon water: Add 2 to 3 slices fresh lemon to water for flavor.

Day 6

GRILLED MARINATED CHICKEN

◆ Toss a 4-ounce chicken breast with 1 tablespoon Italian dressing (like Newman's Own Lighten Up) and 1 tablespoon Parmesan cheese. Cook on a skillet or the grill for 15 to 20 minutes (10 minutes per side) or until the chicken is cooked well.

GRILLED ZUCCHINI

◆ Slice one small zucchini and toss with 1 tablespoon Italian dressing. Sauté in a skillet or on the grill for 7 to 10 minutes or until the zucchini is tender.

WILD RICE

◆ Prepare 1 cup of wild rice (about ⅓ cup of dry rice) per package instructions. Try Lundbery's Brown & Wild Rice Blend or another whole grain blend.

1 cup milk or milk substitute

Snacks & Desserts

Day 1

CHOC-NUTTY BANANAS

INGREDIENTS

1 small banana, sliced

2 teaspoons Nutella (or other nut spread)

DIRECTIONS

◆ Top each banana slice with the Nutella (or other nut spread).

1 ounce part-skim mozzarella cheese stick and a pear

BERRY CREAM FRO-YO DESSERT

Combine ½ cup each fat-free Greek yogurt and mixed frozen berries with 1 packet stevia or 1 teaspoon honey. Blend for 30 seconds using an immersion blender or standing blender. Pour into ice-pop molds if you have them, or just pop the whole bowl into the freezer for 5 to 7 minutes. Eat chilled. Or skip it and spend **150 Flex Calories** however you chose.

Day 2

MINI FRUIT & NUT BAR

(MAKES 32 SERVINGS)

Make your own Fruit and Nut Bars with this recipe from Canyon Ranch, or snack on a similar 100-calorie bar, like KIND Snacks Mini Bars.

INGREDIENTS

½ cup chopped pecans
½ cup chopped almonds
¾ cup honey
2¾ cups rolled oats
½ cup dried cranberries
¾ cup dried chopped apples
½ cup raisins
10 medium-size dates, sliced
1 teaspoon cinnamon

DIRECTIONS

◆ Preheat oven to 325 degrees. Lightly coat a 9-inch by 13-inch baking sheet with canola oil spray. Spread nuts on baking sheet and toast lightly for 5 minutes.

◆ Warm honey in microwave or over low heat on stovetop to the consistency of a thin syrup.

◆ Place nuts in the bowl of a food processor. Chop briefly. Add oats, cranberries, apples, raisins, dates and cinnamon. Turn on machine and chop briefly until all ingredients are chopped. While machine is running, drizzle in warm honey until mixture binds.

◆ Place fruit and nut mixture on baking sheet. Lightly spray parchment paper with canola oil, and place paper over the mixture. Using a rolling pin, roll (over parchment) until mixture is spread evenly. Shape into a rectangle. Place in freezer for at least 30 minutes. Remove from freezer, and cut into 32 mini bars.

TIP: For best results, store wrapped or in an airtight container in the refrigerator for up to 1 month.

Eat with a **small apple**

BLACK BEAN & CORN SALAD

from Jon Rollo of Greenleaf ChopShop

(SERVES 6; 1/2-CUP SERVINGS)

INGREDIENTS

2 ears corn, shucked (about 1 cup)
1 14.5 ounce can black beans, drained and rinsed
1 red bell pepper, diced (about 1 cup)
1 tablespoon minced cilantro
2 tablespoons extra-virgin olive oil
1 tablespoon lime juice
Salt and pepper

TIP: If corn is not in season, substitute fresh for 1 cup frozen corn, thawed.

DIRECTIONS

◆ Cut kernels from corn cobs. In a medium bowl, combine all ingredients. Refrigerate until serving.

150 Flex Calories to spend however you choose.

Day 3

CHIA SEED CHOCOLATE ALMOND MILK

◆ Combine 1 cup dark chocolate almond milk with 1 teaspoon chia seeds.

TIP: Chia seeds absorb 10 times their weight in water. Let this set in the refrigerator for a few hours and the chia seeds will start to absorb some of the liquid and give the drink even more texture.

QUINOA GREEK SALAD

Combine ½ cup cooked quinoa with 2 tablespoons chopped tomato, 2 tablespoons chopped cucumber, ½ teaspoon olive oil, 1 teaspoon balsamic vinegar, ¼ teaspoon garlic powder. Mix and serve.

GRILLED COCONUT CRUNCH PINEAPPLE DESSERT

◆ On a preheated grill, place 4 pineapple slices on a grill screen or in a grill basket. Grill for 3 to 5 minutes on each side until lightly grilled. Serve topped with 1½ tablespoons shredded coconut and 1 teaspoon slivered or chopped almonds. Or skip it and spend **150 Flex Calories** however you choose.

Day 4

BANANA COCONUT SMOOTHIE

◆ Blend together ½ frozen banana with ½ cup light coconut milk. Serve immediately.

CHEESE, CUCUMBER & CRACKER SANDWICHES

◆ Top two Triscuit or Kashi Roasted Garlic crackers with one Laughing Cow Original Creamy Swiss spread (split between the two crackers) and cucumber slices.

150 Flex Calories to spend however you choose.

Day 5

EGG SALAD

◆ Chop one hard-boiled egg with 1 tablespoon light mayonnaise; serve with ½ cup celery sticks.

SAVORY SPINACH BREAD

◆ Toast a slice of whole-wheat bread. In a skillet sauté 1 cup baby spinach until wilted, about 1 to 2 minutes. Then top the toasted bread with the spinach and 3 tablespoons shredded mozzarella cheese. Bake at 350 degrees until the cheese is melted, about 2 to 3 minutes. Finish with ¼ teaspoon garlic powder.

150 Flex Calories to spend however you choose.

Day 6

TRAIL MIX POPCORN

◆ Mix together 1 cup air-popped pop-corn, 1 tablespoon dried cranberries, and 1 tablespoon chocolate chips.

1 ounce whole-wheat pretzels and 2 teaspoons peanut butter

150 Flex Calories to spend however you choose.

WEEKLY AVERAGE DAILY NUTRITION FACTS: 1,500 calories plus 150 Flex Calories for 1,650 calories total, 45 g total fat, 14 g saturated fat, 0 g trans fat, 12 g monounsaturated fat, 5 g polyunsaturated fat, 235 mg cholesterol, 1,594 mg sodium, 203 g carbohydrates, 32 g fiber, 82 grams sugar, 88 g protein. Ratio of calories from carbohydrates, protein, and fat: 56% carbo-hydrates, 21% protein, and 23% fat.

CHAPTER FIFTEEN

HOT & HEALTHY WORKOUT PLANS

STICK WITH THESE ROUTINES TO TONE UP FAST!

Cosmo's team of celebrity trainers have designed these simple exercise plans to score you a sexy, strong bikini body. Get ready to sweat it out and slim down.

This chapter features an easy-to-read recap of each of your workouts in the form of a monthly cheat sheet, followed by detailed week-by-week instructions revealing exactly how to do all the moves. Each week includes:

◆ A fresh Morning Cardio Blast suggestion to keep you from getting bored!
◆ Illustrated moves for the toning routines from Tracy Anderson
◆ Step-by-step directions on how to do the calorie-torching, muscle-building routines specially created for you by the trainers at Barry's Bootcamp
◆ Creative suggestions for a fun new way to spend your Feel-Good Fitness days

Remember to plan your two non-consecutive days off every week to give your muscles time to rest and recover for optimum results!

HOT & HEALTHY
WORKOUT CHEAT SHEET

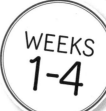

WEEKS
1-4

DAY	WORKOUT	MINUTES
1	Morning Cardio Blast (pages 188, 195, 198, 201)	15
	Tracy Anderson's Toning Routine (pages 188, 196, 199, 202)	6
	TOTAL WORKOUT TIME	**21**
2	Morning Cardio Blast (pages 188, 195, 198, 201)	15
	Barry's Bootcamp Total-Body Strength Circuit (pages 190, 195, 198, 202)	20
	TOTAL WORKOUT TIME	**35**
3	Rest and recover!	
4	Morning Cardio Blast (pages 188, 195, 198, 201)	15
	Tracy Anderson's Toning Routine (pages 188, 196, 199, 202)	6
	TOTAL WORKOUT TIME	**21**
5	Morning Cardio Blast (pages 188, 195, 198, 201)	15
	Barry's Bootcamp Total-Body Strength Circuit (pages 190, 195, 198, 202)	20
	TOTAL WORKOUT TIME	**35**
6	Rest and recover!	
7	Morning Cardio Blast (Optional) (pages 188, 195, 198, 201)	15
	Feel-Good Fitness day (pages 194, 197, 200, 203)	30-45
	TOTAL WORKOUT TIME	**45-60**

MORNING CARDIO BLAST
from Barry's Bootcamp

REPEAT 3 TIMES FOR A 15-MINUTE WORKOUT

JUMP ROPE
2 ½ MINUTES

◆ Use a light standard rope or one with weighted handles for an extra edge.
◆ Land on both feet or alternate feet.
◆ If you have trouble jumping rope, keep working at it. You only get better with practice.

ACTIVE RECOVERY: Dance it out (30 seconds)

BURPEE
1 ½ MINUTES

◆ Jump up, reaching for the sky! (It doesn't have to be high, just get those feet OFF that floor!)
◆ Land on soft knees and go *all the way down* until hands are touching the floor.
◆ Kick your legs back, together and at the same time.
◆ Bring your legs back in, and jump back up.
◆ For that added little edge, add a pushup after you kick your legs back.

ACTIVE RECOVERY: Dance it out (30 seconds)

TIGHTEN UP YOUR BUTT
from Tracy Anderson

6 MINUTES

INVERTED SIDE KICK
1 ½ MINUTES

❶ Get on all fours, and rotate your left leg so your knee is turned in and your shin is out to the side. Rest on your right forearm, and bend your left elbow for leverage.

❷ Kick your left leg out to the side, with shoelaces facing front. That's one rep; do 30, and switch legs.

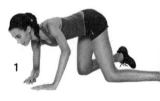

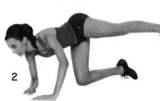

KNEE SWING
1 ½ MINUTES

❶ Begin on your hands and knees, then balance on your left arm and right leg. Bend your left knee, and rest your foot on top of your right ankle; raise your right arm to the side, palm up.

❷ Lift your left leg back and up toward the ceiling. That's one rep; do 30, and switch legs.

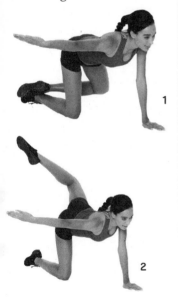

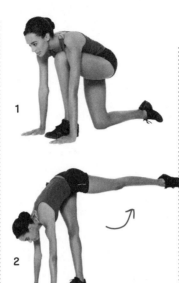

LUNGE AND LIFT
1 ½ MINUTES

❶ Start in a runner's lunge—kneel on your right knee, and place your hands on either side of your left foot.

❷ Straighten your right leg, keep your hands on the floor (move them a few inches forward for more stability), and lift your left leg 90 degrees. That's one rep; do 30, and switch legs.

BUTT BUSTER
1 ½ MINUTES

❶ Get on all fours, then balance on your left arm and left leg (your body will rotate to face the right). Touch your right hand to your left shoulder, and cross your right foot over your left ankle (you'll form a triangle between your legs).

❷ Keep your right knee bent, and raise your leg as high as you can. That's one rep; do 30, and switch legs.

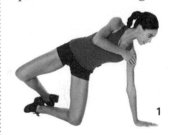

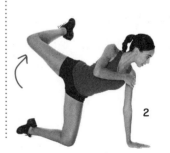

TOTAL-BODY STRENGTH CIRCUIT
from Barry's Bootcamp

20 MOVES IN 20 MINUTES

One circuit means doing each of the four sets of exercise once for the amount of time outline for each exercise. Do the entire circuit once to complete all 20 exercises on this page through 194. Start this week using 5-to 6-pound weights and increase the weight if it feels too easy. Challenge your body for just 20 minutes—then you're done!

SCULPT SEXY ARMS

BICEP CURL
1 MINUTE

◆ Standing with your knees slightly bent, abs in and chest up, hold your arms straight with the palms facing away from you. Watching in the mirror, bring the weights straight up—pretend you are holding a bar in your hands and can't turn your wrists. All the way up and all the way down—don't cheat the distance!

HAMMER CURL
1 MINUTE

◆ Begin with arms straight, palms facing in toward your body.
Don't turn your wrists as you bring them straight up until the weights are right before your shoulders. Lower them back to starting position. Remember to go all the way back down!

TRICEP OVERHEAD EXTENSION
1 MINUTE

◆ Using one dumbbell or two (of course we prefer two if you can), stand or sit while holding the dumbbell(s) by one end above your head (using both hands if you're using only one dumbbell).
◆ Slowly lower the dumbbells until it is hidden behind your head, keeping your elbows in as much as you can.
◆ Press the weights back overhead to return to starting position.
◆ Inhale going down; exhale pushing up.

TRICEP KICKBACK
1 MINUTE

◆ Stand with your feet hip-distance apart, feet parallel, and midsection bent forward with your chest toward the floor. Hold the weights with your palms facing your body.
◆ With your elbows bent and behind you, pull the weights up by your chest. Straighten your arms, pushing the weights all the way back—flex your triceps at the end of each rep.
◆ If you're feeling ambitious, you can turn your palm to face up.

BICEP CURL WITH OVERHEAD EXTENSION
1 MINUTE

◆ Take what you've learned from the bicep curl and tricep overhead extension and combine them.
◆ Standing with your knees slightly bent, abs in and chest up, hold your arms straight with the palms facing away from you. Watching in the mirror, bring the weights straight up—pretend you are holding a bar in your hands and can't turn your wrists. All the way up and all the way down—don't cheat the distance!
◆ Once at the top of the curl, rotate your palms to face one another and use your shoulders to press the weights up overhead.
◆ Slowly lower the dumbbells, until they are hidden behind your head, keeping your elbows in as much as you can.
◆ Press the weights back overhead, and lower to just above shoulders. Rotate your palms to face outward, and slowly lower them back down in the negative bicep curl release.

SCULPT A SEXY CORE

BOXING WITH WEIGHTS
1 MINUTE

◆ We suggest using your lighter set of weights for all phases of this exercise.
◆ Standing with your knees slightly bent, feet hip-distance apart, abs in tight (remember we always work from our core), hold the weights up in front of your chest, under your chin.
◆ Look straight into the mirror and punch 30 seconds with the right arm, then 30 seconds with the left. You should feel your shoulders burning!

STANDING SIDE BEND—WITH OR WITHOUT WEIGHTS
1 MINUTE EACH SIDE OR 2 MINUTES ALTERNATING

◆ We suggest using your heavier set of weights, if you are using any.
◆ Stand with feet shoulder-width apart, knees softly bent, chest up, and eyes forward with abs pulled in and weights by your side. If you elect to do these without weights, place your hands either on top of your head or above your head with fingers interlaced.
◆ Lean as far down as you can to the right, and allow the oblique muscles to pull you back up to standing position.
◆ Repeat on the other side.

JACKKNIFE

30 SECONDS

◆ Use only one dumbbell for this.

◆ Lie on the floor, legs straight and hands cupping the weight behind your head, arms straight.

◆ Bring your head and shoulders up as your arms come up, bringing your arms and legs together as your dumbbell and toes meet over your belly button. If you need to bend your knees a little, that's okay.

PLANK

1 MINUTE

◆ This is one of the best exercises for the core!

◆ Get on your forearms and your toes.

◆ Pull your belly button up into your spine, but breathe!

◆ Hold the position. If you feel like you need a break, stick your booty up in the air instead of letting your knees hit the ground.

◆ Feeling ambitious? Pick up one foot off the ground, keeping the leg straight. Switch legs after a few seconds.

STANDING ROW (FOR YOUR BACK)

1 MINUTE

◆ Stand with your feet hip-distance apart, knees slightly bent. Hold your arms straight with palms facing your thighs.

◆ Bend forward with your chest toward the floor.

◆ Pull up the weights toward you (you can follow your thighs from your knees to your hips). Keep your back straight and bring your shoulder blades together as you bring the weights up. Your elbows should end up behind you at about a 90-degree angle.

◆ Return to starting position by straightening arms, and repeat.

SCULPT A SEXY CHEST & SHOULDERS

CHEST PRESS

1 MINUTE

◆ Lie on the floor with weights in hand and your elbows level with your body at a 90-degree angle, knees bent and feet flat. Tuck your hips.

◆ With palms facing toward your feet and hands right outside your chest,

push the weights all the way up toward each other until they touch directly over your chest. Return to starting position.

◆ Hint: Every day we are asked about the infamous "bra fat." This is the exercise we tell women to focus on!

CHEST FLY

1 MINUTE

◆ More for the "bra-fat" area!

◆ Lie on the floor with your feet flat and knees bent. Tuck your hips.

◆ Start at the top with palms facing each other and weights touching. Lower them slowly toward the floor (never hitting the floor), and bring them back to starting position.

◆ Exhale on the way up; inhale on the way down.

MILITARY PRESS

1 MINUTE

◆ Standing or seated, hold your arms straight out to your sides, elbows level with your shoulders, forearms and palms up—you should look like a goal post!

◆ Slowly push the weights up above your head and toward each other until they gently touch. Watching yourself in the mirror on the way up, imagine a dome on your head—outline that dome with the weights as you go up.

STANDING SHOULDER RAISE
1 MINUTE

◆ Stand with your feet parallel and hip-distance apart with knees slightly bent. Keep your arms straight and palms facing you.

◆ Bring the weights straight up in front of you until they're above your chest, right under your chin—elbows above the shoulders. Lower them down slowly to starting position.

PUSH-UP
30 SECONDS

◆ Feet together or up to 12 inches apart. Your body should be straight all the way down and up. Start and stop in the same position every rep.

◆ Going down, you should break the plane where your shoulders and elbows are parallel. Your arms can be any width that you like—close, shoulder width or even wider, but your hands shouldn't leave

the ground (this means no sliding them to a new position).

◆ Do as many as you can in 30 seconds!

SCULPT A SEXY BUTT AND LEGS

SQUAT
1 MINUTE WITH AN OPTIONAL 30-SECOND RECOVERY BEFORE STARTING THE NEXT EXERCISE

◆ Stand with feet a little wider than hip-distance apart, feet parallel. Hold the weights either at your sides or above your shoulders.

◆ As you lower your booty keep your chest up and all the body weight in your heels.

◆ Go down low as you can, keeping your back straight and chest up.

◆ Always keep your abs tucked in. Inhale going down; exhale coming up.

◆ On the way back up, push your heels into the floor. Remember, your heels never leave the ground.

◆ Return to starting position. Going slow is good—you'll really feel it!

DEAD LIFT
1 MINUTE WITH AN OPTIONAL 30-SECOND RECOVERY BEFORE STARTING THE NEXT EXERCISE

◆ Stand with your feet parallel, hip-distance apart, arms straight holding the weights in front of your thighs, palms facing in.

◆ Knees can be bent (which may help any lower-back issues) or kept straight (to target the hamstrings more).

◆ Bending at the waist, lower the weights slowly until they pass your knees. If you are flexible and want that extra stretch go down lower, but always make sure your back stays straight.

◆ With your abs tight, slowly raise back up to starting position. At the top, tuck and squeeze your butt for that added little edge we love so much.

STATIONARY LUNGE

30 SECONDS ON EACH LEG WITH AN OPTIONAL 30-SECOND RECOVERY BEFORE STARTING THE NEXT EXERCISE

◆ Stand with your feet together, arms straight at your sides holding the weights, palms facing in.
◆ Left foot should stay on the floor where it is.
◆ Lunge far forward with your right foot. You want to be sure to have your foot go far enough so your knee doesn't pass your toes.
◆ Your back knee bends, going as close to the floor as possible.
◆ Keep your abs in, back straight, and chest up.
◆ Return to starting position.

REVERSE LUNGE

30 SECONDS ON EACH LEG WITH AN OPTIONAL 30-SECOND RECOVERY BEFORE STARTING THE NEXT EXERCISE

◆ Stand with your feet together, arms straight at your sides holding weights and palms facing in.
◆ Left leg should stay put—right foot goes as far behind as you as you're able, as you bend the left knee.
◆ Keep your abs in, back straight, and chest up.
◆ Return to start position.

PLIÉ SQUAT

1 MINUTE

◆ Don't worry—you won't need ballet shoes for this move, but it does target your butt nicely for sculpted dancer's limbs.
◆ Stand with feet wide, toes out pointing away from each other (think east and west), and hold weights above your shoulders.
◆ Keeping your chest up and back straight, lower yourself slowly toward the ground by bending your knees, back straight. Your heels should be glued to the floor with knees going toward the toes but never beyond them.
◆ Return to starting position.
◆ For an added burn, try holding or pulsing at the bottom.

FEEL-GOOD FITNESS
MAKE YOUR SWEAT SESSION A MASH-UP

Switch things up and do about 45 minutes of some type of exercise that feels fun, such as playing basketball, or else one that feels relaxing, such as yoga or Pilates. You might just want to sign up for a weekly class, like a karate, Zumba, or swim class, if these are workouts you really enjoy. Or maybe you'd rather just get outside and power walk (you should be too out of breath to hold a conversation) or jog for your Feel-Good Fitness day. It's totally up to you!

One celeb fitness-class trend to watch: FitMix classes in Los Angeles, which were created by trainer Diana Newton. The enviably sculpted star of CBS's *2 Broke Girls*, Beth Behrs, swears by them—they call for 25 minutes of supersweaty cardio intervals followed by 30 minutes of muscle-quivering Pilates moves. "The intervals burn crazy calories while the Pilates changes your body to give you a long and lean look," says Newton.

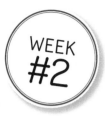

MORNING CARDIO BLAST
from Barry's Bootcamp

REPEAT 3 TIMES FOR A 15-MINUTE WORKOUT

SHADOW BOX

1 ½ MINUTES

◆ Time to get in touch with your inner Rocky!
◆ Face the mirror. Your feet should be constantly moving side to side as you box.
◆ Keep your fists up, and punch either straight forward or crossing right to left.
◆ Add some upper cuts for fun. Just don't stop moving!

ACTIVE RECOVERY: WALL SIT
(30 seconds)

◆ Lean against a wall with your knees bent at 90-degree angles and your back straight.

HIGH KICK

1 MINUTE

◆ Keep your right leg stable as your left leg kicks high up in front of you for 30 seconds. Keep the leg your're standing on soft— no locked knees!
◆ Switch to the other leg and repeat for 30 seconds.

ACTIVE RECOVERY: WALL SIT
(30 seconds)

MOUNTAIN CLIMBER

1 ½ MINUTES

◆ Place your hands on the floor, shoulder-width apart.
◆ Your shoulders should be directly over your hands.
◆ Your legs should be straight out behind you.
◆ Don't let your booty go too far up in the air as you do this—keep it level as possible!
◆ Bring one knee quickly into your chest before bringing it straight out behind you again into starting position. As soon as your leg is straight back, bring the opposite

knee into your chest. Keep quickly alternating your knees to your chest for a killer cardio move.
✦ Remember to move as fast as you can!

TOTAL-BODY STRENGTH CIRCUIT
from Barry's Bootcamp

20 MOVES IN 20 MINUTES

Repeat the 20 moves on page 190 through page 194 using 5-to 6-pound weights. Do one set of the entire circuit (or 20 exercises total).

TONE UP THREE TIMES FASTER
from Tracy Anderson

6 MINUTES

LEG AND ARM RAISE

1½ MINUTES

❶ Begin on your hands and knees, gripping a 20-ounce water bottle in your right hand. Extend your right leg straight behind you, toes touching the ground.

❷ Lift your right leg to hip height (your shoelaces should face out) while raising your right arm. That's one rep; do three sets of 10, and change sides.

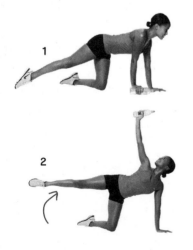

REACH AND TWIST

1½ MINUTES

❶ Start in a lunge, with your left knee on the ground and your right leg bent 90 degrees. Grip the bottle in your right hand, and reach past your toes.

❷ Rotate your torso and right leg to the left, so your right knee drops to the floor (your left leg and knee will naturally pivot). At the same time, reach your right arm toward the ground. That's one rep; do three sets of 10, and switch sides.

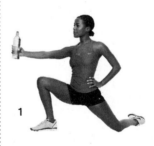

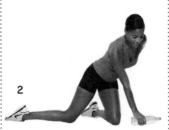

PLANK PUSH-BACK

1½ MINUTES

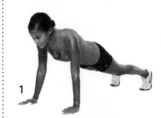

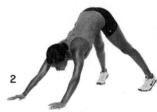

❶ Begin in a plank—legs and back straight, belly tight. Hold for three seconds.

❷ Push back into downward dog: Lift your tailbone to the ceiling, keep your arms and legs straight, and press your heels toward the ground. Hold for three seconds. That's one rep; do three sets of 10.

SIDE BRIDGE KICK

1 ½ MINUTES

1 Lie on your left side, elbow underneath your shoulder, and lift your hips so your upper body makes a straight line. Extend your right leg to the front, a few inches off the ground, toes pointed.

2 Kick your right leg back and up, slightly higher than your hips. That's one rep; do three sets of 10, and switch legs.

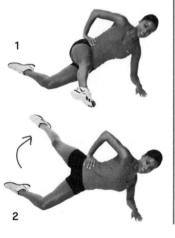

1

2

FEEL-GOOD FITNESS
TRY A NEW FUSION CLASS

Do something today that you enjoy and that moves your body—such as power walking outside.

For something different, check out a Core Fusion class, which could be a mix of yoga, Pilates, ballet, and strength training. Exhale Spas feature Core Fusion Cardio, Core Fusion Boot Camp, Core Fusion Sport, Core Fusion Yoga, and more. Go to ExhaleSpa.com to find a class near you.

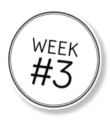

WEEK #3

MORNING CARDIO BLAST
from Barry's Bootcamp

REPEAT 3 TIMES FOR A 15-MINUTE WORKOUT

JUMP SQUAT
2 MINUTES

◆ You don't have to jump high—just get your feet off the floor, but jump as high as you are able to. And you don't have to go all the way down—just land in a squat with your knees slightly bent when you land.

◆ *Don't land on a straight leg!* Always keep knees soft on landing.

ACTIVE RECOVERY:
Plié squats
(30 seconds)

◆ Stand with your feet wide and your toes out pointing away from each other (think east and west).

◆ Keeping your chest up and back straight, lower yourself slowly toward the ground by bending your knees. Your heels should be glued to the floor, with your knees going toward the toes but never beyond them.

◆ Return to starting position.

KNEE RAISE
1 MINUTE

◆ Stand on the right leg, soft knee—lean forward, chest toward the floor.

◆ *Quickly* bring the left knee toward the chest and back to the floor.

◆ After 30 seconds switch legs.

◆ You can use arm motions with the hands to help with balance and add some cardio effect.

✦ Remember to keep your abs tight and in!

ACTIVE RECOVERY: Plié squats (30 seconds)

BURPEE
1 MINUTE

◆ Jump up, reaching for the sky! (It doesn't have to be high, just get those feet *off* that floor!)

◆ Land on soft knees and go *all the way down* until hands are touching the floor.

◆ Kick you legs back, together at the same time.

◆ Bring your legs back in, and jump back up.

◆ For that added little edge, add a push-up after you kick your legs back.

TOTAL-BODY STRENGTH CIRCUIT
from Barry's Bootcamp

20 MOVES IN 20 MINUTES

◆ Repeat the 20 moves on page 190 through page 194, but this week challenge your body by upping your weights to 8 pounds. Do all 20 exercises once, challenging your body for just 20 minutes—then you're done!

SLIM YOUR WAIST
with Tracy Anderson

MINUTES

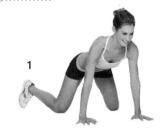

1

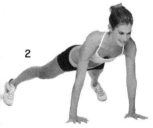

2

WIDE LEG PLANK

½ MINUTES

❶ Start on your hands and knees, legs slightly wider than hip-width apart. Your arms should be directly under your shoulders, abs tight.

❷ Raise up into plank position: knees off the floor, legs and back straight, belly pulled in. Hold for a few seconds, and lower down to start. That's one rep; do three sets of 10.

SIDE BRIDGE

1 ½ MINUTES

❶ Lie on your right side, with your right arm underneath your shoulder and legs stacked.

❷ Tighten your core, and lift your hips so your body makes a diagonal line. Hold for a few seconds, and return to start. That's one rep; do three sets of 10, and switch sides.

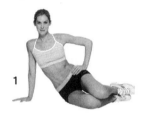

1

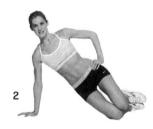

2

BELLY TWISTER

1 ½ MINUTES

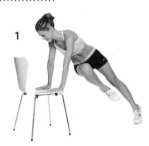

1

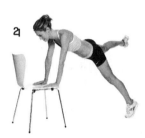

2

❶ Begin in plank pose, with your palms placed on the seat of a chair. Lift your right knee in toward your abs, and twist it to the left, so your outer thigh is parallel to the chair.

❷ Extend your right leg back 90 degrees on the diagonal. Return to start, with the knee pulled toward your core. That's one rep; do three sets of 10, and change legs.

V CRUNCH

1 ½ MINUTES

1 Start in a basic crunch, with your feet flat on the floor, knees bent, hands behind your head, and shoulders lifted a few inches.

2 Extend and lift both legs off the floor (your right leg should rise only a few inches), and cross your left leg over your right. Return to start. That's one rep; do three sets of 10, and switch sides.

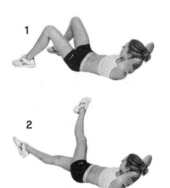

FEEL-GOOD FITNESS

TEST OUT THE CROSSFIT TREND

It's your day to move your body in any way that feels good or to try doing something totally new. If you haven't yet joined the CrossFit trend, you might want to test it out. Stars like Jessica Biel and Jessica Alba are big fans of this supereffective but hardcore workout. Cameron Barden, a coach at CrossFit 212, in New York City, explains how you can benefit from it too.

First Timer? You may have heard about the intense WOD (workout of the day). But don't let that scare you off. Most CrossFit gyms have a beginner's class, often called Foundations, that slowly introduces you, over the course of six sessions, to the moves that make up all of CrossFit's routines. **No Bulk.** CrossFit works your entire body at once and burns major calories, so you'll end up strong and toned. And FYI, you won't get superjacked like the women on Reebok's CrossFit Games (those tough ladies do way more than CrossFit a few times a week).

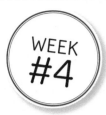

WEEK #4

MORMING CARDIO BLAST
from Barry's Bootcamp

REPEAT 3 TIMES FOR A 15-MINUTE WORKOUT

FAST FEET & DROP SQUAT

1 MINUTE

◆ Move your feet in front of you, going back and forth as fast as you can as if you're tapping your toes.

◆ Bend your knees and keep your abs in, chest up, and back straight. You're in a semisquat.

◆ Count! Every five seconds, drop down to the lowest squat possible and pop right back up!

◆ In class, we yell "drop" every time you need to squat...so you've been spared that luxury.

ACTIVE RECOVERY: Boxing Shuffle (30 seconds)

◆ Stand with your arms up covering your face, like a boxer, and shuffle your feet from side to side.

CROSS MOUNTAIN CLIMBER

1 MINUTE

◆ Place your hands on the floor, shoulder-width apart. Your shoulders should be directly over your hands.

◆ Your legs should be straight out behind you.

◆ Don't let your booty go too far up in the air as you do this—keep it as level as possible!

◆ *Slowly* alternating your legs, bring the knee to the opposite elbow.

◆ This is great for your core—keep your abs up and tight, and breathe!

◆ Don't worry if you stop during the minute—just get back into it. Do as much as you can in the minute you have!

ACTIVE RECOVERY: Boxing Shuffle (30 seconds)

JUMPING JACK

2 MINUTES

◆ This one may take you back to childhood, but it's tried and true!

◆ Remember to stay on the balls of your feet and keep your knees *soft*—not locked.

◆ Hands touch at the top *every time*.

◆ Adding a clap at the top guarantees you touch every time and adds that little extra edge we love so much.

TOTAL-BODY STRENGTH CIRCUIT
from Barry's Bootcamp

20 MOVES IN 20 MINUTES

Repeat the 20 moves on page 190 through page 194, sticking to your heavier, 8-pound weights. Do all 20 exercises once. Challenge your body for just 20 minutes—then you're done!

LEAN THIGHS— NO LUNGES!
with Tracy Anderson

KARATE KICK

1 ½ MINUTES

1 Start in a squat, with both legs bent 90 degrees (don't let your knees extend past your toes) and your feet turned out. Use the chair for balance.

2 Come out of the squat, and kick your left leg to the side at hip height, foot flexed and facing forward. That's one rep; do three sets of 10, and switch legs.

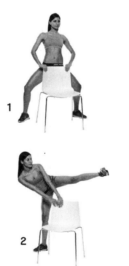

DIAGONAL LIFT

1 ½ MINUTES

1 Stand on your left leg, hands on the chair, and extend your right leg behind you, toes on the floor. Turn out your right leg so your shoelaces face the side.

2 Bend and lift your leg above hip height—keep your toes pointed, and rest your left hand on the seat. That's one rep; do three sets of 10, and change sides.

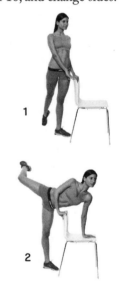

LEG EXTENSION
1½ MINUTES

1 Lift your right leg, knee bent 90 degrees and toes pointed, so your thigh clears the back of the chair and your toes hover above the seat.

2 Extend your leg behind you, rotating it out so your shoelaces face the side. That's one rep; do three sets of 10, and change sides.

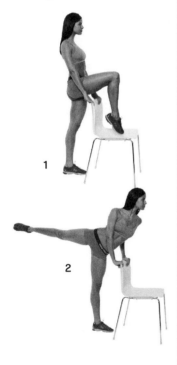

SIDE RAISE
1½ MINUTES

1 Stand, feet parallel, with your right hand on the chair and your left hand on your hip. Pull your belly in toward your spine.

2 Lift your left leg straight out to the side, about 45 degrees, toes pointed. Your shoelaces should face forward. That's one rep; do three sets of 10, and switch sides.

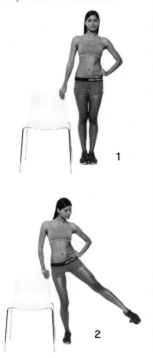

FEEL-GOOD FITNESS
RUN FOR YOUR LIFE!

You're on the tail end of your first month of the Cosmo Bikini Diet, so try something different today to keep your workouts feeling fresh. An idea: the zombie workout. Nothing like being chased by a mob of the undead to get you sprinting. Zombies, Run! is an audio app for your smartphone that guides you through heart-pumping zombie apocalypse missions, and the only way to escape is to keep running. Once you've survived, compare your mileage and pacing stats on the app's website.

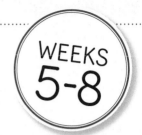

HOT & HEALTHY
WORKOUT CHEAT SHEET

WEEKS
5-8

DAY	WORKOUT	MINUTES
1	Morning Cardio Blast (pages 205, 209, 212, 215)	15
	Tracy Anderson's Toning Routine (pages 207, 210, 213, 216)	6
	TOTAL WORKOUT TIME	**21**
2	Morning Cardio Blast (pages 205, 209, 212, 215)	15
	Barry's Bootcamp Rubber Band Workout (pages 205, 209, 212, 215)	25
	TOTAL WORKOUT TIME	**40**
3	Rest and recover!	
4	Morning Cardio Blast (pages 205, 209, 212, 215)	15
	Tracy Anderson's Toning Routine (pages 207, 210, 213, 216)	6
	TOTAL WORKOUT TIME	**21**
5	Morning Cardio Blast (pages 205, 209, 212, 215)	15
	Barry's Bootcamp Rubber Band Workout (pages 205, 209, 212, 215)	25
	TOTAL WORKOUT TIME	**40**
6	Rest and recover!	
7	Morning Cardio Blast (Optional) (pages 205, 209, 212, 215)	15
	Feel-Good Fitness day (pages 209, 211, 214, 217)	30-45
	TOTAL WORKOUT TIME	**45-60**

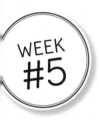

MORNING CARDIO BLAST
from Barry's Bootcamp

15 MINUTES

Time to run it out! Do this on a treadmill, a track, a park with a big field, or on the road in front of your house.

◆ 3-minute walking or light jog warm-up
◆ 1-minute run
◆ 1-minute sprint (*go for it!*)
◆ 1-minute recovery (you've earned it)
◆ 2-minute run
◆ 1-minute sprint
◆ 1-minute recovery
◆ 30-second sprint
◆ 30-second recovery
◆ 2-minute speed walk
◆ 1-minute jog
◆ 1-minute sprint
◆ *Recover!*

RUBBER BAND WORKOUT
from Barry's Bootcamp

25 MINUTES

You'll start with a lighter resistance band for weeks 5 and 6, and as you become used to the routine, you'll switch to a heavier one for weeks 7 and 8 (see page 11 for details on how to choose the right resistance band for you). Remember, using strong resistance bands that challenge your body will give you more defined, faster results! Give yourself a 30-second active recovery (think: jogging in place, jumping jacks, or dance it out) between each exercise, and do this 8-move exercise circuit twice for a total-body toning workout in only about 25 minutes!

SQUAT
1 MINUTE

◆ Stand with your feet a little bit wider than hip-distance apart with the band securely beneath each foot.
◆ Hold the handles in each hand, right above your shoulders.
◆ Chest up and abs in, keeping your feet glued to that floor!
◆ Slowly lower your butt but don't go past your knees.
◆ Slowly return to starting position.
◆ Remember, these are resistance bands, so move slowly and use that resistance.

RUBBER BAND DANCE!

LENGTH OF SONG, APPROXIMATELY 2 MINUTES

◆ Time for some real fun. Pick out your favorite song. (We suggest something with a cool groove, maybe a hip-hop beat like "Bootylicious" Rockwilder Remix!)

◆ Stand on the band, feet a little bit more than hips distance apart.

◆ Cross the band handles creating an X with the band.

◆ Pull the handles up above your hips and hold them there

◆ Now step side to side in time with the music. Here's where we find out who's got rhythm.

◆ Do the whole song. Make sure you have attitude like "yeah, my butt's firm."

LEG EXTENSIONS

1 MINUTE

Okay so everything may not be as fun as the rubber band dance but in the name of firm thighs and butt, we will do anything! Well, almost anything…

◆ Fit the handles over the toe of your sneakers.

◆ Lie on the ground with the band under your butt—hands will be under there holding the band in place.

◆ Head and shoulders just lay against the ground, knees bent (tabletop position)

◆ Slowly straighten your legs out, flexing the quad muscles.

◆ Slowly return to starting position.

◆ You can do both legs for one minute or each leg for 30 seconds.

INNER-THIGH EXTENSION

1 MINUTE

◆ Stay down on the ground with the band and hands exactly as they were for during leg extensions.

◆ Now straighten your legs and point your toes away from you (toes to the ceiling).

◆ Spread your legs apart as far as you're able to, and bring them back together.

◆ It's a scissor motion. Engage your inner thighs on the way in.

BUTT LIFTS

2 MINUTES

◆ With one of the band handles wrapped securely around one foot, get on all fours—forearms and knees.

◆ Hold the band in the same hand as the foot you have the band on.

◆ Bring your knee up off the floor and push the leg straight back all the way, making sure it's tight so there is tension. Your foot should be above your booty, creating about a 90-degree angle.

◆ One minute on each leg—it's worth it!

BICEP CURL

1 MINUTE

◆ Stand on the band with your feet parallel and hip-distance apart.

◆ Your arms should be straight, palms facing out.

◆ Curl the band all the way up, with your forearms moving toward the bicep.

◆ Squeeze at the top every time.

MILITARY PRESS

1 MINUTE

◆ Stand on the band with your feet parallel hip-distance apart and your knees slightly bent.

◆ Hold the bands above your shoulders, palms facing out.

◆ Push the handles up and overhead.

◆ For an added edge, you can do a squat and over-head combo.

SHOULDER RAISE

1 MINUTE

◆ Stand on the band with your feet hip-distance apart and knees slightly bent.

◆ Your arms should be straight, palms facing in. Pull the band up.

◆ Lead with your elbows. Hands come above the chest right under the chin, and your elbows are above your shoulders.

◆ Return to start position.

◆ For that added some-thing, you can step side to side while bringing the band up and down and get some butt in there while your shoulders burn!

CELLULITE-ZAPPING WORKOUT
with Tracy Anderson

6 MINUTES

LUNGE KICK

1 ½ MINUTES

❶ Begin in a lunge, with your right knee bent and your left leg extended back, knee and toes on the floor. Plant your hands on the ground inside your right knee, elbows straight.

❷ Kick your right leg be-hind you, shoelaces facing the side, foot flexed. Then return to start. That's one rep; do three sets of 10, and switch legs.

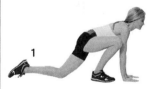

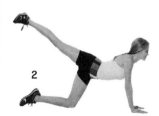

BUTT LIFT
1½ MINUTES

❶ Lie on your stomach, with your legs bent (your knees should be wider than hip distance) and heels touching. Lift your upper chest off the floor, resting on your forearms.

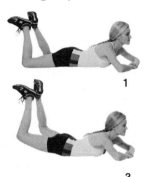

❷ Squeeze your butt to raise your legs a few inches, then lower back to start. That's one rep; do three sets of 10.

CRISSCROSS
1½ MINUTES

❶ Sit on the ground, feet planted in front of you and hands on the floor behind you (arms straight, fingers facing your butt). Lift your hips, and cross your right leg over your left.

❷ Straighten your right leg, and lower it to the right so the outside of your shoe touches the ground. Pause for a second or two, then cross it back over the left leg. That's one rep; do three sets of 10, and change sides.

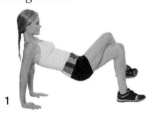

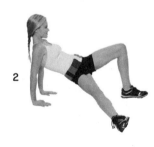

BOOTY PUSH
1½ MINUTES

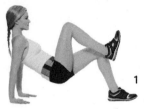

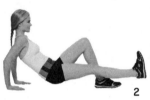

❶ Start in the same beginning position as the Crisscross, but this time, raise your right leg (keep your knee bent), and flex your foot.

❷ Extend your right leg, bend your elbows, and lower your butt so it's a few inches off the floor. That's one rep; do three sets of 10, and switch legs.

FEEL-GOOD FITNESS
POUND IT OUT!

By now you've probably been experimenting with at least a few of the creative new workout trends suggested for these Feel-Good Fitness days. This week, you might try rocking out with a total-body cardio routine created by recreational LA drummers Kirsten Potenza and Cristina Peerenboom, who combined their love of music with fitness to create the POUND workout.

The moves are a cross between drumming, Pilates, and the Bar Method, and you'll swap hand weights for weighted drum sticks to get toned all over. If you're curious, you can stream classes on your laptop or mobile device with the Backstage Pass online subscription at PoundFit.com. It gets you a set of Ripstix and a 1-month membership for $14.99 for the first month, and then if you like it, you pay $9.99 each month after. The creators feature a new music-driven workout every week so you don't get bored.

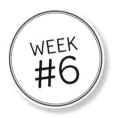

WEEK
#6

MORNING CARDIO BLAST
from Barry's Bootcamp

REPEAT 3 TIMES FOR A 15-MINUTE WORKOUT.

CROSSOVER HOP
2 MINUTES

◆ Lay a jump rope on the floor in a straight line.

◆ Place your hands on the floor shoulder-width apart, with the jump rope in between your hands.

◆ With your feet together, keep your hands on the floor and hop over the rope (bend your knees here!).

◆ If you get tired doing this, hold position for a few and get back in it.

ACTIVE RECOVERY: Plié Squats (30 seconds) (see page 198 for instructions)

HIGH KICK
2 ½ MINUTES

◆ Keep your right leg stable as left leg kicks high up in front of you. Keep the leg you're standing on soft—no locked knees! (30 seconds)

◆ Switch to the other leg (30 seconds).

◆ Repeat on each leg for a total of two times.

ACTIVE RECOVERY: Plié Squats (30 seconds)

RUBBER BAND WORKOUT
from Barry's Bootcamp

25 MINUTES

◆ Repeat the routine on page 205 using your lighter resistance band. Give yourself a 30-second active recovery between each exercise, and do this 8-move exercise circuit twice for a total-body toning workout in only 25 minutes!

LOWER-BODY BLAST
with Tracy Anderson

6 MINUTES

KNEELING SIDE EXTENSION
1 ½ MINUTES

1 Grab a (very solid!) chair. Carefully position your left knee and shin on the chair seat, with its back to your left. Grip the chair back with your left hand. Slowly bend your right knee, and hover your right foot in front of the seat while resting your right hand on your hip.

2 Slowly lift your right arm to shoulder height and your right leg to hip height. Straighten and extend both away from your body. Return to start. That's one rep; do 30, and switch sides.

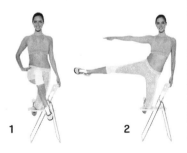

BETTER-BOOTY KICK
1 ½ MINUTES

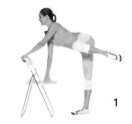

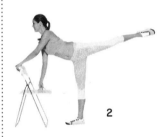

1 With your feet a few inches behind the chair, grip its back with your left hand and the edge of the seat with your right hand. Keeping your right leg straight, raise your left leg to hip level and turn it out, bending to 90 degrees.

2 Straighten and extend your left leg directly behind you, as though you are kicking something. Return to start. That's one rep; do 30, and switch sides.

STANDING TOE KICK
1 ½ MINUTES

1 Hold the chair back for support with your right hand. Anchor your right foot behind the chair, and place your left foot on the chair seat while raising your left arm to shoulder height and extending it away from your body.

2 Raise your left foot, and point your toe as you kick it forward, straightening your leg. Return to start. That's one rep; do 30, and switch sides.

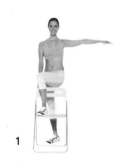

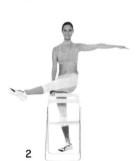

LEANING CHAIR CRUNCH

1 ½ MINUTES

1 Sit near the edge of the chair seat with feet wider than shoulder-width apart. Grasp the chair at hip height for support. Bending from your hips, lean your chest forward.

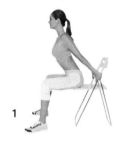

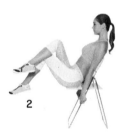

2 Move your hand grip to the chair's legs and lift feet; bend knees and slowly rock back into the seat. Cross your right knee over your left knee, and return to start. That's one rep; do 30, and switch sides.

FEEL-GOOD FITNESS

TRY THE TRAMPOLINE WORKOUT!

Trampoline classes are popping up in gyms across the country, where you get a workout by getting your bounce on. It's great cardio that improves your balance all while feeling like child's play—especially if you're moving up and down to your favorite playlist. If your local gym doesn't offer trampoline classes, you can try getting your own and setting up in your living room for a fun way to fit in some commercial cardio while watching your favorite shows. Jump Sport sells a fitness trampoline that comes with a basic fitness DVD (jumpsport.com).

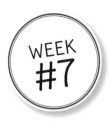

MORNING CARDIO BLAST
from Barry's Bootcamp

REPEAT 3 TIMES FOR A 15-MINUTE WORKOUT

MOUNTAIN CLIMBER

1 MINUTE

◆ Place your hands on the floor, shoulder-width apart. Your shoulders should be directly over your hands.

◆ Your legs should be straight out behind you.

◆ Don't let your booty go too far up in the air as you do this—keep it as level as possible!

◆ Bring one knee quickly into your chest before bringing it straight out behind you again to starting position. As soon as your leg is straight back, bring the opposite knee into your chest. Keep quickly alternating your knees to your chest for a killer cardio move.

◆ Remember to move as fast as you can!

ACTIVE RECOVERY: Slow jog (30 seconds)

KNEE RAISE

1 MINUTE

◆ Stand on the right leg, with a soft knee—lean forward chest toward the floor.

◆ *Quickly* bring the left knee toward the chest and back to the floor.

◆ After 30 seconds, switch legs.

◆ You can use arm motions with the hands to help with balance and add some cardio effect.

◆ Remember to keep your abs tight and in!

ACTIVE RECOVERY: Slow jog (30 seconds)

MOUNTAIN CLIMBER

2 MINUTES

◆ Repeat, as above.

RUBBER BAND WORKOUT
from Barry's Bootcamp

25 MINUTES

◆ Repeat the routine on page 205 switching to your heavier resistance band. Give yourself a 30-second recovery between each exercise, and do this 8-move exercise circuit twice for a total-body toning workout in only 25 minutes!

GET A TIGHT, SEXY CORE
with Tracy Anderson

6 MINUTES

SUPERWOMAN PLANK

1½ MINUTES

1 Begin in a plank position, with your legs split wide.

2 Extend your left arm forward and right leg back, and pull your core into your spine. Keep the hip bones angled toward the floor, and don't let them open as the leg extends. That's one rep; do 30, and switch sides.

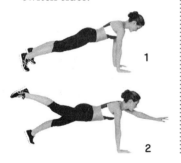

TORSO TWISTER

1½ MINUTES

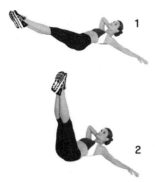

1 Start on your back with legs stretched straight out and angled to the left side, about 45 degrees off the ground. Hold your left arm behind your head with the right arm extended out to the right side for balance.

2 Lift legs up to 90 degrees. That's one rep; do 30, and switch sides.

CROSS-LEG CRUNCH

1½ MINUTES

1 Lie on your back with your hands behind your head and torso crunched up. Stretch out your legs so they're a few inches off the floor and your right ankle is crossed on top of your left.

2 Pull your legs into your chest, keeping your ankles crossed. That's one rep; do 30, and switch your top leg.

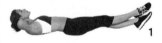

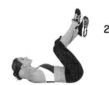

SIDE-LUNGE EXTENSION

1 ½ MINUTES

1 Start in a plank position with your hands placed underneath your shoulders. Bring your right leg into a side lunge, making sure to stay on the ball of your right foot.

2 Extend your right leg diagonally back, lifting it higher than your butt. That's one rep; do 30, and switch sides.

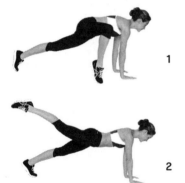

1

2

FEEL-GOOD FITNESS

ROCK A MUD RUN

The dirtiest fitness craze starts with a fun run, then adds actual fun: Friends, crazy obstacles, and post-race beers. Sign up for a mud run at LoziLu.com. Just avoid these newbie mistakes:

◆ **I don't need to train.** You'll enjoy race day more if you're in shape. Do a few pre-event jogs on grass, and stop every couple of minutes to do push-ups, crunches, and squats.

◆ **I'll wear a bikini.** Just as you wear supportive sneaks, a sports bra would be wise.

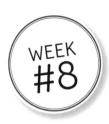

MORNING CARDIO BLAST
from Barry's Bootcamp

REPEAT 3 TIMES FOR A
15-MINUTE WORKOUT.

JUMP ROPE

2 MINUTES

◆ Using either a light
standard rope or one with
weighted handles for an
extra edge.
◆ Land on both feet or
alternate feet.
◆ If you have trouble
jumping rope, keep work-
ing at it. You only get
better with practice.

ACTIVE RECOVERY:
Boxing Shuffle
(30 seconds)
◆ Stand with your arms
up covering your face, like
a boxer, and shuffle your
feet from side to side.

BURPEE

2 MINUTES

◆ Jump up, reaching for
the sky! (It doesn't have to
be high, just get those feet
off that floor!)
◆ Land on soft knees and
go *all the way down* until
hands are touching the
floor.
◆ Kick your legs back,
together, and at the same
time.
◆ Bring your legs back in,
and jump back up.
◆ For that added little
edge, add a push-up after
you kick your legs back.

ACTIVE RECOVERY:
Boxer Shuffle
(30 seconds)

RUBBER-BAND WORKOUT
from Barry's Bootcamp

25 MINUTES

◆ Repeat the routine on
page 205, sticking to your
heavier resistance band.
Give yourself a 30-second
recovery between each
exercise, and do this
8-move exercise circuit
twice for a total-body
toning workout in only 25
minutes!

SHAPE SEXY ABS, SUPERFAST!
with Tracy Anderson

6 MINUTES

◆ All these exercises use a chair, which provides extra stability. As a result, it's easier for you to focus on tightening your core so you get more out of each move.

WAIST SHRINKER

1½ MINUTES

❶ Sit on the edge of a chair with your left leg crossed over your right. Rest your right arm on the back of the chair, and extend your left arm straight up.

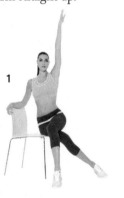

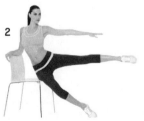

❷ Lift your left leg out to the side at hip height, shoelaces facing the front. Lower your left arm to the side, palm facing down. That's one rep; do 30, and switch sides.

BENT-KNEE CRUNCH

1½ MINUTES

❶ Lie on your back, and grip the legs of a chair behind you (it should be about 6 inches away from your head). Lift your feet 6 inches off the floor.

❷ Tighten your abs to pull both legs in, bending your knees and keeping the soles of your feet together. That's one rep; do 30.

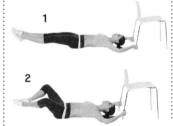

SINGLE-LEG LIFT

1½ MINUTES

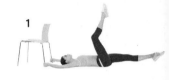

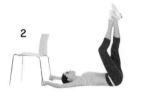

❶ Lie flat on your back while holding onto a chair, but this time, lift your right leg 90 degrees, with your knee bent. Keep your left leg straight out in front of you, and raise it 6 inches off the floor.

❷ Lift your left leg up to meet your right leg, so your right ankle touches your left. That's one rep; do 30, and switch legs.

TUMMY TUCK

1½ MINUTES

1 Start in the same position as the Bent-Knee Crunch.

2 Lift both legs 90 degrees, toes pointed, and lower back down to start. That's one rep; do 30.

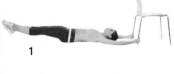

1

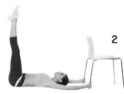

2

FEEL-GOOD FITNESS

FIND YOUR FITNESS INSPIRATION

If you're looking for more exercise-idea inspiration, *Jillian Michaels: Hard Body* DVD will kick your ass in all the right ways ($15, collagevideo.com). But sometimes the hardest part is actually pushing play. Jillian gets it. Her advice: "Skip generalizations like 'I want to be healthy.' Get specific to find real, lasting motivation. Is it skinny jeans? Sex with the lights on? Spring break? More energy?"

HOT & HEALTHY WORKOUT CHEAT SHEET

WEEKS 9-12

DAY	WORKOUT	MINUTES
1	Morning Cardio Blast (pages 219, 222, 225, 228)	15
	Tracy Anderson's Toning Routine (pages 220, 223, 226, 229)	6
	TOTAL WORKOUT TIME	**21**
2	Morning Cardio Blast (pages 219, 222, 225, 228)	15
	Barry's Bootcamp Total-Body Strength Circuit—Times Two! (pages 219, 223, 225, 228)	40
	TOTAL WORKOUT TIME	**55**
3	Rest and recover!	
4	Morning Cardio Blast (pages 219, 222, 225, 228)	15
	Tracy Anderson's Toning Routine (pages 220, 223, 226, 229)	6
	TOTAL WORKOUT TIME	**21**
5	Morning Cardio Blast (pages 219, 222, 225, 228)	15
	Barry's Bootcamp Total-Body Strength Circuit—Times Two! (pages 219, 223, 225, 228)	40
	TOTAL WORKOUT TIME	**55**
6	Rest and recover!	
7	Morning Cardio Blast (Optional) (pages 219, 222, 225, 228)	15
	Feel-Good Fitness day (pages 221, 224, 227, 230)	30-45
	TOTAL WORKOUT TIME	**45-60**

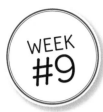

WEEK
#9

MORNING CARDIO BLAST
from Barry's Bootcamp

REPEAT 3 TIMES FOR A 15-MINUTE WORKOUT

FAST FEET & DROP SQUAT
1 MINUTE

◆ Move your feet in front of you, going back and forth as fast as you can as if you're tapping your toes.

◆ Bend your knees and keep your abs in, chest up, and back straight. You're in a semisquat.

◆ *Count!* Every 5 seconds, drop down to the lowest squat possible and pop right back up! In a class we yell "drop" every time you need to squat...so you've been spared that luxury.

ACTIVE RECOVERY:
Dance it out
(30 seconds)

CROSS MOUNTAIN CLIMBER
1 MINUTE

◆ Place your hands on the floor, shoulder-width apart. Your shoulders should be directly over your hands.

◆ Your legs should be straight out behind you.

◆ Don't let your booty go too far up in the air as you do this—keep it as level as possible!

◆ *Slowly* alternating your legs, bring the knee to the opposite elbow.

◆ This is great for our core—keep your abs up and tight, and breathe!

◆ Don't worry if you stop during the minute—just get back into it. Do as much as you can in the minute you have!

ACTIVE RECOVERY:
Dance it out
(30 seconds)

SHADOW BOX
2 MINUTES

◆ Time to get in touch with your inner Rocky!

◆ Face the mirror; feet should be constantly moving side to side as you box.

◆ Keep your fists up and punch either straight forward or crossing right to left.

◆ Add some upper cuts for fun. Just don't stop moving!

TOTAL-BODY STRENGTH CIRCUIT
from Barry's Bootcamp

20 MOVES IN 20 MINUTES—TIMES TWO!

◆ Repeat the 20 moves on page 190 through page 194, but this time try using heavier, 10-pound weights. Do one set of the entire circuit (or 20 exercises total) and then repeat for a total of two sets. Challenge your body for just 40 minutes—then you're done!

UPPER-BODY BLAST
with Tracy Anderson
6 MINUTES

KNEELING HAND PRESS
1½ MINUTES

❶ Begin on all fours with two 3-pound weights in your left hand, palm facing away from your body. Keep your right arm straight with palm flat on the ground. Maintain a slight bend in your left elbow.

❷ Bend through your left elbow to push and extend left arm straight up to the ceiling, keeping your gaze at a fixed point on the ground and your neck relaxed. Return arm to floor; that's one rep. Do 30, and switch arms.

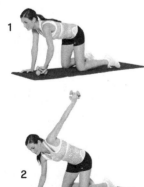

LASSO ARM
1½ MINUTES

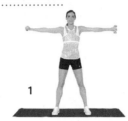

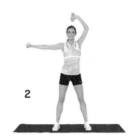

❶ Hold a weight in each hand. Extend both arms straight out from your sides like a T, with right palm down and left palm facing the back wall.

❷ Bend left arm at the elbow, and swing it up and forward, holding the weight about six inches above your head, palm facing forward. Swing your arm back to starting position, with palm facing backward. That's one rep; do 30, and switch arms.

ELBOW RAISE
1½ MINUTES

❶ Kneel with legs shoulder-width apart. Secure weights in your right hand. Hold right arm across your body at a 90-degree angle. Hold weights in front of your belly button, palm facing up. Extend your left arm, keeping your hand 12 inches from your leg.

❷ Raise weights to chest level, flipping palm outward and reaching your right elbow out at a diagonal. That's one rep; do 30, and switch arms.

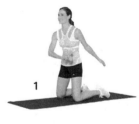

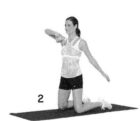

SINGLE-ARM V PRESS

1½ MINUTES

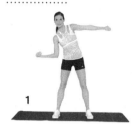

1 Hold a weight in each hand, and extend left arm straight out to the left side of your body. Bend your right arm at the elbow, crunching in your obliques and creating a 90-degree angle, palm facing up.

2 Press right arm up and away from the body, with palm reaching toward ceiling. That's one rep; do 30, and switch arms.

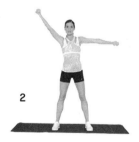

FEEL-GOOD FITNESS
PLAY A GAME AGAINST YOURSELF

Make your workout more fun by turning it into a sort of competition against yourself with a heart rate monitor. Gym goers at the new Momentum fitness studio in Santa Monica, California, are getting fitter faster by wearing Polar Cardio GX heart rate monitors during classes, such as CrossFit Yoga. "This makes it easy to hit your target heart rate zones to maximize your results and motivates you by showing exactly how many calories you burned during your class," says Jennifer Cohen, owner of Momentum and trainer on the former CW show *Shedding for the Wedding*.

Challenge yourself to stay in the zone by wearing your own heart rate monitor to gauge if you're exercising at your target heart rate or if you need to increase or decrease your intensity. "It makes your time at the gym much more efficient," says Cohen. "It also counts your calories more accurately than machines, and the Polar heart rate monitors are super easy to use. I end up wearing mine all day." (Polar heart rate monitors start around $59; amazon.com).

"Wearing a heart rate monitor turns exercise into a game when you push yourself to stay within your heart rate zone or to burn more calories than you did last time," says Cohen. You should aim to be between 65 and 90 percent of your target heart rate. To find yours, subtract your age from 220 and then multiply that number by .75 (to be at 75 percent). For example, if you're 25 years old, your number would be about 146 beats per minute. If you're doing interval training, you'd want to alternate between the low end of your heart rate and the high end (90 percent) to burn the most calories and get the fastest results.

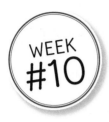

MORNING CARDIO BLAST
from Barry's Bootcamp

REPEAT 3 TIMES FOR A 15-MINUTE WORKOUT.

FAST FEET & DROP SQUAT
1 MINUTE

◆ Move your feet in front of you, going back and forth as fast as you can as if you're tapping your toes.

◆ Bend your knees and keep your abs in, chest up, and back straight. You're in a semisquat.

◆ *Count!* Every 5 seconds, drop down to the lowest squat possible and pop right back up! In class we yell "drop" every time you need to squat...so you've been spared that luxury.

ACTIVE RECOVERY:
Dance it out
(30 seconds)

CROSS MOUNTAIN CLIMBERS
1 MINUTE

◆ Place your hands on the floor, shoulder-width apart. Your shoulders should be directly over your hands.

◆ Your legs should be straight out behind you.

◆ Don't let your booty go too far up in the air as you do this—keep it as level as possible!

◆ *Slowly* alternating your legs, bring the knee to the opposite elbow.

◆ This is great for your core—keep your abs up and tight, and breathe!

◆ Don't worry if you stop during the minute—just get back into it. Do as much as you can in the minute you have!

ACTIVE RECOVERY:
Dance it out
(30 seconds)

SHADOW BOX
2 MINUTES

◆ Time to get in touch with your inner Rocky!

◆ Face the mirror; feet should be constantly moving side to side as you box.

◆ Keep your fists up and punch either straight forward or crossing right to left.

◆ Add some upper cuts for fun—just don't stop moving until the time is up!

TOTAL-BODY STRENGTH CIRCUIT
from Barry's Bootcamp

20 MOVES IN 20 MINUTES—TIMES TWO!

◆ Repeat the 20 moves on page 190 through page 194, using 10-pound weights. Do one set of the entire circuit (or 20 exercises total) and then repeat for a total of two sets. Challenge your body for just 40 minutes—then you're done!

THREE SLIMMING WORKOUTS IN ONE
with Tracy Anderson

6 MINUTES

KNEE PLANK

1½ MINUTES

❶ Kneel on all fours with your knees hip-distance apart. Use your right arm for support, and wrap a towel around your left calf. Your body should make a straight line from your knees to your head.

❷ Extend your right leg behind you on the diagonal (your torso will naturally lean closer to the floor). That's one rep; do 30, and switch sides.

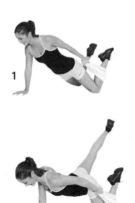

LUNGE AND LIFT

1½ MINUTES

❶ Start on all fours and wrap the towel around your upper right arm, crossing your left arm behind your back to hold on to it. Lunge your left leg forward, and keep your right knee on the ground and your left heel lifted.

❷ Lift your left leg behind you, toes pointed. That's one rep; do 30, and change sides.

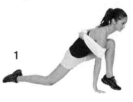

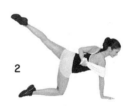

CRUNCH AND REACH

1½ MINUTES

1 Kneel with your legs hip-distance apart. Grip the towel on either end, and lean your torso to the left.

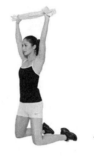

2 Now lean all the way to the right, so your torso is parallel to the floor and your right hand is on the ground for support. Lift your left leg out to the side, just above hip height. That's one rep; do 30, and switch sides.

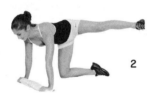

KNEELING KICK

1½ MINUTES

1 Kneel with your legs hip-distance apart and arms extended straight above your head, holding the towel taut on both ends.

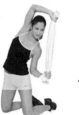

2 Lower your hands to the floor so you're on all fours, and kick your left leg out to the side. That's one rep; do 30, and change sides.

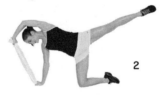

FEEL-GOOD FITNESS

MIX UP YOUR ROUTINE

Hitting the same gym for the same workout every time you exercise gets boring fast... and can fizzle your results. Check out FITiST.com, a website that allows you to try fun, new classes at the buzziest boutique studios for a set fee, without paying for a membership at the fancy venues you check out. Sample Pilates near your office Monday morning, do Spinning by your apartment Wednesday night, and box in your BF's hood on Saturday afternoon. The site is rolling out in 10 cities and counting.

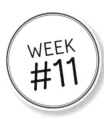

MORNING CARDIO BLAST
from Barry's Bootcamp

REPEAT 3 TIMES FOR A
15 MINUTE ROUTINE

KNEE RAISE

1 MINUTE

◆ Stand on the right leg, soft knee. Lean forward with your chest toward the floor.

◆ *Quickly* bring the left knee toward the chest and back to the floor.

◆ After 30 seconds switch legs.

◆ You can use arm motions with the hands to help with balance and add some cardio effect.

◆ Remember to keep your abs tight and in!

ACTIVE RECOVERY:
Stationary lunges
(30 seconds)

◆ Stand with your feet together, arms straight at your sides holding the weights, palms facing in.

◆ Your left foot should stay on the floor where it is.

◆ Lunge far forward with your right foot. You want to be sure to have your foot go far enough so your knee doesn't pass your toes.

◆ Your back knee should bend, going as close to the floor as possible.

◆ Keep your abs in, back straight, and chest up!

◆ Return to starting position. Alternate legs.

JUMP SQUAT

1 MINUTE

◆ You don't have to jump high—just get your feet off the floor, but jump high as you are able to. And you don't have to go all the way down—just land in a squat with your knees slightly bent when you land.

◆ *Don't land on a straight leg!* Always keep knees soft on landing.

ACTIVE RECOVERY:
Stationary lunges
(30 seconds)

HIGH KICK

1 MINUTE

◆ Keep your right leg stable as left leg kicks high up in front of you. Keep the leg your're standing on soft—no locked knees!

◆ After 30 seconds switch legs.

TOTAL-BODY STRENGTH CIRCUIT
from Barry's Bootcamp

20 MOVES IN 20
MINUTES—TIMES TWO!

◆ Repeat the 20 moves on page 190 through page 194, and keep your weights to your heaviest set at 10 pounds (go for 12-pounds if you're feeling really diesel). Do one set of each of the exercises (or 20 exercises total) and then repeat it again for a total of two entire circuits. Challenge your body for just 40 minutes—then you're done!

YOUR BUTT, ONLY BETTER
with Tracy Anderson
6 MINUTES

HIP DROP AND KICK
1½ MINUTES

❶ Kneel on all fours with knees together, palms under shoulders and arms straight. Supporting yourself with your right arm, drop your right hip to the floor. Lift your hip and rotate your body into start position, but don't let your right knee touch the floor, and balance on your left forearm.

❷ Kick your right leg up to the ceiling. Return to kneeling start position; that's one rep. Do 5 to 20 reps on one side, and switch sides.

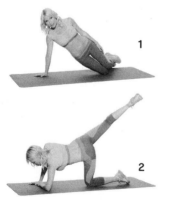

ATTITUDE PULSE
1½ MINUTES

❶ Kneel on all fours with knees together. Balancing on your right forearm and right knee, lift your bent left leg so your thigh is at hip height. Lift your leg a few inches, pause, then lower to hip height.

❷ Raise your leg a few inches, then fully extend your leg up toward the ceiling. Then lower to hip height; that's one rep. Do 5 to 20 reps on one side, and switch sides.

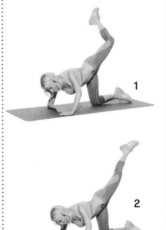

HIP DIP WITH LIFT
1½ MINUTES

❶ Start in plank position with arms straight. Balance on the ball of your left foot, and lift your bent right leg until your thigh is just above hip height.

❷ Rotate your torso to lower your right hip so your knee touches the floor; try to get your entire right outer thigh to touch the floor. Return to plank position; that's one rep. Do 10 to 20 reps on one side, and switch sides.

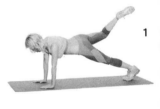

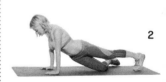

KNEELING BUTT LIFTER

1½ MINUTES

1 Start in kneeling position. Position your forearms under your chin so they're touching, and balance on them. Raise your left foot to create a 45-degree bend in your knee, and swing your foot out a few inches to activate more muscles.

2 Extend your right foot up toward the ceiling so your leg is straight (don't just kick it behind you). Touch your knee to the floor; that's one rep. Do 20 to 50 reps on one side, and switch sides.

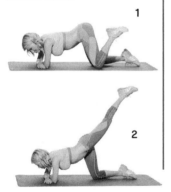

FEEL-GOOD FITNESS DAY

TAKE IT OUTSIDE

Enjoying your exercise more may be as easy as going green: Just five minutes of outdoor activity boosts your mood, finds researchers at the University of Essex in the U.K. If you're a treadmill addict, try doing hills in the park. Rollerblading, biking, and surfing are just a few outdoor exercise alternatives. Or join an outdoor softball, soccer, tennis, or other league at Active.com.

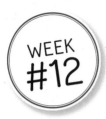

MORNING CARDIO BLAST
from Barry's Bootcamp

REPEAT 3 TIMES FOR A 15-MINUTE WORKOUT

HOPPING OVER THE ROPE

2 MINUTES

◆ Lay your jump rope on the floor in a U-shape. Make the U as wide as you can handle it… You see this coming…

◆ Jump over the U shape—both feet at the same time.

◆ Remember to go as fast as you can—you are aiming to get your heart rate up.

◆ If you need to alternate feet and jump one at a time that's ok. Just keep moving!

ACTIVE RECOVERY:
Jumping Jacks
(30 seconds)

◆ This one may take you back to childhood, but it's tried and true!

◆ Remember to stay on the balls of your feet and keep your knees *soft*—not locked.

◆ Hands touch at the top *every time*.

◆ Adding a clap at the top guarantees you touch every time and adds that little extra edge we love so much.

JUMP SQUAT

1 MINUTE

◆ You don't have to jump high—just get your feet off the floor, but jump high as you are able to. And you don't have to go all the way down just land in a squat with your knees slightly bent when you land.

◆ Don't land on a straight leg! Always keep knees soft on landing.

ACTIVE RECOVERY:
Jumping Jacks
(30 seconds)

RUNNING IN PLACE
1 MINUTE

◆ It is as simple as it sounds except…make sure to bring your knees up as high as you can.

◆ For that extra little edge, hit each knee, opposite hand to knee as you bring them up.

◆ If the high knees get too challenging, just keep running in place until you catch your breath.

TOTAL-BODY STRENGTH CIRCUIT
from Barry's Bootcamp

20 MOVES IN 20 MINUTES—TIMES TWO!

Repeat the 20 moves on page 190 through page 194, sticking to your heaviest, 12-pound weights. Do one set of the entire circuit (or 20 exercises total) and then repeat for a total of two sets. Challenge your body for just 40 minutes—then you're done!

WHOA, NICE ABS!
with Tracy Anderson

6 MINUTES

SIDE-TO-SIDE SIZZLE

1½ MINUTES

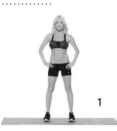

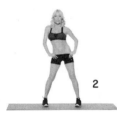

❶ Start with your hands on your hips, standing with your feet just wider than hip-width apart. Your hips should be square, and your toes should face forward.

❷ Keeping your legs firmly planted and your hips stationary, shift your ribs to the right, then back to the left. That's one rep; do 30.

FOLD-OVER WAIST WHITTLER

1½ MINUTES

❶ Start in the same position as the move above.

❷ With your back straight, fold over at your waist, until your head is at hip level and you're looking at the floor. Then lift yourself back to start.

❸ Keeping your legs firmly planted and your hips stationary, shift your ribs to the right and return to start. Repeat step 2, then shift hips to the left. That's one rep; do 30.

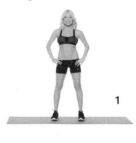

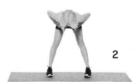

ABS SHIMMY

1½ MINUTES

❶ Start by standing with feet just wider than shoulder-width apart, arms extended overhead, and hands clasped, palms facing ceiling. There will be a slight arch in your lower back.

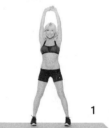

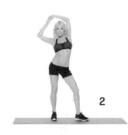

❷ Twist on your left foot to thrust your right hip out as you bend your arms and lower your right elbow toward your right hip. Return to start. That's one rep; do 30, and switch sides. Tip: Arching your lower back a bit gets your core muscles going and helps engage the obliques.

PLIÉ PENDULUM
1½ MINUTES

❶ With your hands resting on your hips, squat with feet just wider than shoulder-width apart, toes at 45-degree angles, and thighs as close to parallel with the floor as possible.

❷ Push off your heels to stand up. Turn in from your ankle until your right toe faces forward, and extend your straightened right leg out to your side, until it's at least a foot off the floor. That's one rep; do 10 to 20, and switch sides. Bonus for your backside: This move works your hamstrings and glutes to lift and tone your butt.

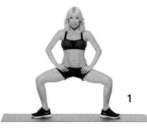

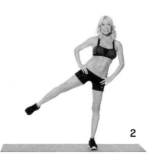

FEEL GOOD FITNESS
PADDLEBOARDING

Take a break from the gym and fit in a workout at the beach by trying something new, like paddleboarding. Imagine combining surfing with kayaking and you've got SUP, the fastest growing water sport in the world. "It's an amazing full-body workout that improves your core strength, cardio fitness, balance, and flexibility with virtually no impact," says Cody White, certified PaddleFit instructor and co-founder of Finger Lakes Paddleboard.

Unlike surfing, you don't need waves to paddleboard. While very calm, flat water is best for beginners, you can do it on an ocean, lake, or even a river. The World Paddle Association (WPA) makes it easy to find races, meet-ups, and classes across the country.

To get started for yourself, White suggests taking a lesson. "The key to mastering paddleboarding isn't about how strong you are, but rather it's all about technique," says White. To avoid common beginner mistakes (think: standing looking down rather than gazing ahead at the horizon for better balance), paddleboarding newbies should sign up for a lesson from a PaddleFit- or WPA-certified instructor. An intro class will show you how to correctly size and hold a paddle, proper paddling technique, basic turns on the board, how to stay safe in wind and waves, and how to fall and remount.

METRIC CONVERSION CHART

VOLUME

USA	CANADA
1 teaspoon	5 ml
1 tablespoon	15 ml
¼ cup	60 ml
⅓ cup	80 ml
½ cup	120 ml
⅔ cup	160 ml
¾ cup	180 ml
1 cup	240 ml
1 pint (U.S.)	475 ml
1 quart	.95 liter
1 quart plus ¼ cup	1 liter
1 gallon (U.S.)	3.8 liters

TEMPERATURE

(To convert from Fahrenheit to Celsius: subtract 32, multiply by 5, then divide by 9)

USA	CANADA
32°F	0°C
212°F	100°C
250°F	121°C
325°F	163°C
350°F	176°C
375°F	190°C
400°F	205°C
425°F	218°C
450°F	232°C

WEIGHT

USA	CANADA
1 ounce	28.3 grams
4 ounces	113 grams
8 ounces	227 grams
12 ounces	340.2 grams
1 pound	.45 kilo
2 pounds, 3¼ ounces	1 kilo (1,000 grams)

INDEX

ABOUT THE AUTHOR AND CONTRIBUTORS

HOLLY C. CORBETT writes for many national women's magazines and is the co-author of a memoir called *The Lost Girls*. She is the founder of the charity race called Runaway Bridesmaids, in which women and men race in recycled bridesmaids' dresses to raise money to fight sex trafficking.

MOLLY MORGAN, RD, CDN, CSSD is the author of *The Skinny Rules* and *Skinny-Size It* and the owner of Creative Nutrition Solutions. Molly develops recipes and customized meal plans for professional athletes and corporate clients.

TRACY ANDERSON is one of the world's most renowned experts in health and fitness. The Tracy Anderson Method has won clients including Gwyneth Paltrow, Victoria Beckham, Nicole Richie, Courteney Cox, Sienna Miller, Jennifer Lopez, and Bethenny Frankel. Tracy develops new routines constantly to ensure that no client ever plateaus. With four studio locations and multiple DVDs, Tracy has transformed the bodies of thousands of people.

BARRY'S BOOTCAMP With locations throughout California, the East Coast, and internationally, this fitness studio's mission is to provide the best cardio and strength program in one hour's time featuring the most current music and qualified trainers in a fun, party environment. Barry's Bootcamp has become a favorite among celebrities like Kim Kardashian, Jessica Biel, Katie Holmes, and Christina Applegate.

Cover and book design by Jill Armus

Photography Credits
Front and back cover images: Michael Poehlman/Getty Images
Exercise photos pages 189-224: Chris Eckert/Studio D
Exercise photos pages 226-230: Perry Hagopian

ISBN 978-1-936297-69-6
Cataloging-in-Publication Data available from the Library of Congress

10 9 8 7 6 5 4 3 2 1

Published by Hearst Editions/Hearst Magazines
300 West 57th Street
New York, NY 10019

Cosmopolitan is a registered trademark of Hearst Communications, Inc.

www.cosmopolitan.com

Distributed to the trade by Hachette Book Group

All US and Canadian orders:
Hachette Book Group
Order Department
Three Center Plaza
Boston, MA 02108
Call toll free: 1-800-759-0190
Fax toll free: 1-800-286-9471

For information regarding discounts to corporations,
organizations, non-book retailers and wholesalers;
mail order catalogs; and premiums, contact:
Special Markets Department
Hachette Book Group
237 Park Avenue
New York, NY 10017
Call toll free: 1-800-222-6747
Fax toll free: 1-800-222-6902

For all international orders:
Hachette Book Group
237 Park Avenue
New York, NY 10017
Tel: 212-364-1325
Fax: 800-364-0933
international@hbgusa.com

Printed in the USA